HOMEOPATHY

Beyond Flat Earth Medicine

D0167906

HOMEOPATHY

Beyond Flat Earth Medicine

An Essential Guide for the Homeopathic Patient

Timothy R. Dooley, N.D., M.D.

Timing Publications

San Diego

Editing: Paul Bergner
Typography and design: Kamala Otee and Ming Dooley
Cover layout and design: Kamala Otee
Cover art: Tim Dooley

ISBN 1-886893-00-4
Library of Congress Catalogue Card Number: 95-60000

Publisher's Note:
The ideas, procedures, and suggestions contained in this book are
not intended as a substitute for consulting with your physician.

See back page for ordering information.

Acknowledgments

Thanks to the following for their reading of the initial manuscripts, helpful comments, or other contributions: Lynne Smith, Kamala Otee, Martin Bloch, M.D., Dennis Gay, Marnie Vail, M.D., Tanya Kell, Katherine Dublinski, Jade Biagioni, John Collins, N.D., Carol Bloch, Jacquelyn Wilson, M.D..

Special thanks to my wife, Ming, for her help in every phase of this project.

Dedication

To my children:
Eamon, Shane, Conan, and Brennan,
who,
along with my wife, Ming,
create the home in
homeopathy.

"The Phlat Earth"
Illustration by Eamon Dooley

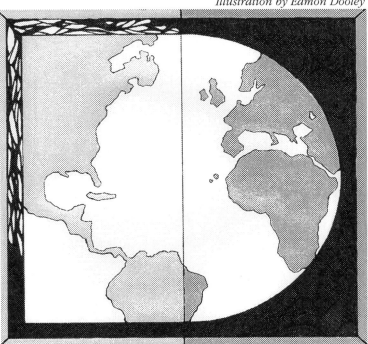

One who drew it, One who never saw it, One who understood it, and One who wanted to eat it.

Contents

Preface

For years my patients have asked me, "What book do you recommend I read to learn about homeopathy?"

Despite an abundance of books on the subject, there was no single book which I felt sufficiently explained the concepts and information needed.

So, I wrote one. This book is based on my own experiences and observations, which over the years have confirmed the basic theories of homeopathy.

Few people really "get it" when they are first introduced to homeopathy. The concepts are straightforward, yet somehow elusive. People attempt to understand and interpret homeopathy based on their prior education and experience. This is only natural, but will limit their ability to perceive something truly different.

Most physicians foolishly reject homeopathy, despite the fact that they know nothing about it. After all, how valid can it be if they, the experts, were not taught about it in medical school?

Homeopathy, however, stands on its own. Its increasing popularity and use suggests that all healthcare providers, whether or not they agree with homeopathy, should at least be familiar with its basic tenets and those who practice it responsibly.

Chapter 1

Beyond the Flat Earth

I had just opened my naturopathic practice in 1978 when a 25-year-old nursing mother entered my office.

Her complaint was mastitis, a painful infection of the breast. The problem had begun some five or six weeks earlier. She had just completed her second course of antibiotic therapy from her medical doctor. Each time the antibiotics ran out, the problem would recur with a vengeance. She had continued to breast-feed throughout the ordeal.

The patient was in a great deal of pain. She said it felt as if the pain radiated from her breast throughout her whole body.

She had a fever with a temperature of around 101 F. On examination her right breast showed an angry red streak extending along its side. It was very tender to touch.

I took her case according to the homeopathic system and prescribed a medicine for her. It was the homeopathic remedy known as Phytolacca 30C.

I was inexperienced at that time in treating complaints of this nature. I knew this could turn into a much worse condition, such as breast abscess, and thought perhaps she really should be on antibiotics. But she was fed up with the antibiotic approach and insisted on trying the remedy.

I told her to call the office first thing in the morning and report how she was doing. She agreed and went on her way.

That night I lay awake in bed with anxiety. I suspected it had been irresponsible for me to treat this patient homeopathically. I feared she had already taken a turn for the worse and perhaps was at the hospital emergency room.

The next morning when I arrived at the office, I pulled her chart and called her without waiting to see if she would report in as agreed.

She was surprised to receive a call from her doctor.

"How are you doing today?" I inquired.

"I'm fine," she said. "The pills worked."

"What do you mean 'the pills worked'?" I asked.

"Well, I mean they worked. It's all gone."

"You mean, the infection is all well, the fever and everything?" I asked, unable to hide my incredulity.

"Yes, it's all fine . . . isn't that what was supposed to happen?"

"Er, ah, why yes, of course that was what was supposed to happen. I was just checking up," I replied, regaining my professional composure. I told her to stop taking the medicine, and to call me if there was any recurrence.

From that moment, I gazed on my little white homeopathic globules with new found respect. I had not thought it was possible for such an infection, with such an acute presentation, to completely disappear overnight. On one dose of the remedy!

When I saw her a month or so later during a visit for her child, she told me the infection had started to come back about a week after the remedy, so she had taken a second dose and everything stayed well after that.

This kind of remarkable cure becomes more common as one gains experience in homeopathic prescribing. The secret is individualizing, treating each patient as a unique whole.

The whole earth view

Few people today would argue that the earth is flat. Everyday experiences such as satellite television and airplane travel all attest to the simple fact that the earth is a sphere.

But it wasn't always so. Even to this day, because of its enormous size, the earth appears flat to the earthbound observer. We still refer to the end of the day as the sunset, indulging in the illusion that it is the sun which has moved behind the visible horizon.

In the past, people were taught from birth that the earth was flat. Science, religion, and common sense all combined to reinforce this perspective. It is easy to appreciate the great conflict that arose among these people when new theories of a spherical earth suggested that their world view was inaccurate. It was impossible for those clinging to the flat view to appreciate the spherical perspective as long as flat thinking was used in its evaluation.

As such, those advocating the spherical earth appeared to be talking nonsense. You could see the earth was flat, that the sun moved across the sky, that things fell down, that water lay flat. All the existing technologies, and there were many, had been developed on a flat world and worked beautifully (they still do today!).

Eventually this conflict was resolved when the flat view was understood to be encompassed within the more comprehensive spherical view. The flat view works to a point, but is only a limited perspective of the same spherical earth.

A new perspective in medicine

A conflict as basic as the flat earth versus spherical earth has existed in the world of medicine for the past 200 years. At that time, a new theory was advanced by a German physician, Samuel Hahnemann. His theory represented a radical departure from the accepted view of health and disease.

Hahnemann proposed that disease is a process that affects the patient as a whole and that medicines can be applied in small, non-toxic doses to treat the patient directly instead of just treating the disease. For reasons which will be explained, he called this new system of medicine *homeopathy*.

Conventional medicine continues to take the older approach. The diseases are treated, not the patient. In fact, *the concept of treating the patient directly, as opposed to the disease, does not even exist!*

To this day, conventional medicines are still classified according to the diseases which they treat. For example, anti-inflammatories treat inflammation, anticonvulsants treat convulsions, and antibiotics kill bacteria.

The idea of a medicine directly treating a patient is quite different from this disease approach. The basic idea is that the medicine stimulates the natural recuperative processes of the patient towards health. The disease resolves naturally as the patient recovers. The disease is not being directly treated and so, for a given disease, there are hundreds of medicines which might be indicated. It depends on the patient. Likewise, for a given medicine, there are hundreds of diseases in which it might be indicated. It depends again on the patient.

Surprisingly, these ideas are as new to most of us now as they were 200 years ago when first formulated. Yet homeopathy is a highly developed science and is used throughout the world.

Flat-earth medicine

Conventional medicine is "flat earth" in that it approaches health problems from the perspective of the disease instead of the patient. Just as the earth appears flat and the sun appears to revolve around the earth, so also it appears that physicians are treating patients when treating their diseases. *This is not true!* As you will see, it is possible to treat the patient directly, as a whole.

As you progress through this book, you'll see how the homeopathic approach to the patient is more comprehensive and encompasses the conventional disease approach in much the same way as the spherical earth view encompasses the flat view. Just as the technologies which developed on the flat earth continue to work and be used today, so also the disease treatments that have developed work fine . . . but only within the disease perspective.

And just as the spherical earth can not be understood as long as flat thinking is used in its evaluation, so also homeopathy makes little sense if only conventional medical thinking is used in trying to understand it. A new perspective is required — a perspective you will get from this book.

After graduating from National College of Naturopathic Medicine in 1978, I spent a number of years in my naturopathic practice in southern Oregon. I gained much firsthand experience in many facets of natural healing. With my partner and two midwives, I ran a home birth program and delivered babies both in town and in homes out in the woods. Using spinal manipulation, I treated mill workers with sore backs. Some of my patients received nutritional therapy, and many benefited from the herbs which grew in the surrounding forests and fields.

But my first love was always homeopathy. I used it in patients young and old for conditions as simple as colds, as chronic as arthritis, and as acute as infections. I learned that all types of healing and healthcare have a place, but homeopathy has a special place. It is safe, yet effective, and is based on clear principles.

The reactions of the local medical doctors to our presence were varied. Some were respectful, but wary, while others were openly antagonistic. "It's against medical ethics for me to even talk to you!" an ophthalmologist once screamed at me over the phone.

These doctors did not seem to share our conviction that all forms of healing have a place, that it all depends on the needs of the patient.

The shortcomings of the disease approach

Everyone today knows that there have been benefits from the conventional disease approach to healthcare. Deadly diseases of the past, such as pneumonia, are treated routinely with great success. But consider the following discussions between the imaginary Dr. Smith and a few of his patients.

#1 "I'm sorry, Mrs. Jones. All my tests indicate you are in perfect health."

"But Dr. Smith, I feel terrible so much of the time. Isn't there something else we can do?"

"Well, sometimes a trial course of antidepressants is helpful."

Disease model problem: If the disease cannot be diagnosed, there can be no treatment.

This is a much bigger problem than would appear on the surface.   First of all, most patients have had various symptoms for years before a diagnosable problem arises. They are told to use one drug or another for symptomatic relief until finally a definitive diagnosis can be made.

It should be obvious that the patient was sick long before the disease could be diagnosed. People have symptoms because something is wrong, but modern medicine, with almost pathological egotism, dares to tell people they are fine when they do not feel well.   Does conventional medicine know everything? Of course not. When they say, "Everything is fine, it must be in your head," what they should be saying is, "We can't identify a known disease diagnosis for your complaints."

Even if a diagnosis is made, it isn't necessarily correct. Various studies have determined that diagnoses made by physicians are correct only around fifty to seventy five per cent of the time. The disease treatment for an incorrectly diagnosed problem obviously will be of little help and may be quite harmful.

#2   "Dr. Smith, Jimmy has been coughing for three weeks! Isn't there something we can give him?"

"Jimmy's lab tests indicate this is a viral syndrome and antibiotics are not effective against viruses. However, if you like, we could try a course and see if it helps."

Disease model problem: For many diagnosable conditions, no treatment exists.

Once again, this is a much bigger problem than it might appear on the surface. At least Dr. Smith has been honest in acknowledging the treatment will probably be of little value. Unfortunately conventional physicians routinely over-diagnose and over-treat many complaints. In such situations, the patient gets well in spite of the treatment, not because of it.

#3　"This is Carol's fifth ear infection this year, Dr. Smith. The medicine is costing $75 per course. Isn't there something we can do to prevent this from recurring?"

"Well, perhaps a course of low dose antibiotics in between infections will help. If not, I'll give you a referral to a specialist for the placement of tubes in the ears."

Disease model problem: Treatment for recurring problems does little to prevent future incidents.

Health problems recur due to continued susceptibility in the patient, but the disease approach rarely addresses this susceptibility. Each recurrence is treated as if it is a new problem resulting in a revolving-door experience for the patient: treatment, recurrence, treatment, recurrence, etc.

Dr. Smith is probably a sincere individual doing his best to help the patients. Yet the above scenarios represent only a fraction of the limitations of the disease model in healthcare. Consider the further problems of drug side effects and adverse reactions. Consider the terrible problem of increasing bacterial resistance to antibiotics due to their overuse.

Consider the cost of healthcare. The disease model requires the development of increasingly sophisticated technologies to diagnose diseases with greater certainty. A few patients certainly benefit, but most are merely undergoing increasingly expensive evaluations that find nothing or discover that they have a disease where no satisfactory treatment exists.

When this disease model is promoted as the only viable avenue to healthcare it becomes more than just a disease model — it becomes flat-earth medicine. It becomes a fixed view that blinds one to the benefits of any other perspective.

There have been many benefits through the development of the disease-oriented view. Homeopathic physicians have, from the beginning, recognized the need for surgery, nutrition, and other modalities. But the flat-earth approach of using medicines only to treat diseases, not patients, is of limited value and carries a much greater risk than many people currently recognize.

Chapter 2

The Basics of Homeopathy

As the years went by, I decided to return to conventional medical school. There was no single reason for this, I loved naturopathic medicine and homeopathy. I did want to learn more about such things as emergency medicine and surgery and I felt more training would make me a better doctor. But perhaps more than this was the desire to see what it was like from the other side, to see if I was missing something that conventional medicine had. I wanted to see if medical doctors really had some kind of special knowledge to justify their superior attitude, some knowledge to which I was not a party.

My time as a student at Oregon Health Sciences University School of Medicine passed quickly. The first two years were the basic science years. I was accustomed to these from naturopathic medical school and they were mostly review to me. The second two years were mostly hospital work, doing rotations in various specialities such as surgery, pediatrics, and psychiatry.

As the time passed, I began to realize that something was indeed missing, not with me, however, but with conventional medicine! It lacked an underlying perspective or basis in approaching patients. There was no real appreciation for the ability of the body to heal itself. The patient's diseases were treated, often with love and caring, but there was not even a concept of working with the natural recuperative powers of the patient. Patients were treated as broken biochemical machines.

I learned a great deal in my medical training and met many fine people, but the wonder and enchantment of natural healing were nowhere to be found. I came to realize that no conventional medical specialty could satisfy me, that I would return to homeopathy.

The law of similars

The practice of homeopathy is based on an observation called the *law of similars.* What this means, in simple terms, is that what a substance can cause, it can cure.

For example, Hahnemann's initial experiments were with Cinchona bark, from which quinine is derived. He found that if it is given in daily doses to a healthy person it can cause symptoms similar to malaria. Indeed, this same Cinchona is curative in many patients with malaria.

There are many examples of this principle of "like cures like." Everyone knows how coffee keeps people awake and alert. In homeopathy it is used in very small doses to cure patients with just that same kind of insomnia associated with an overly alert mind.

The name *homeopathy*

As Hahnemann developed this idea of similars into a science he gave it the name *homeopathy.* The Greek roots to this word are *homoios* meaning "similar" and *pathos* meaning "suffering". So the name homeopathy reflects the basic theory as well as the mode of treatment. That is, a substance can be used as a medicine when the symptoms that the patient is experiencing are similar to the symptoms that a healthy individual would experience if they were taking that same substance.

Hahnemann also named the conventional system of medicine. Since these doctors give patients substances that cause symptoms different from those they are experiencing, the proper name is *allopathy* (*allo* meaning "other"). The appropriate name for conventional medicine remains allopathic medicine and this term, allopathy, is used at times in this book.

The minimum dose

"Above all do no harm" is an ancient medical maxim which is followed in homeopathy. Hahnemann was faced with the problem of trying to use medicines in such a way that they wouldn't cause more problems. He found that if a medicine was well indicated by its similar symptoms, it could be given in very small doses with excellent results.

Through experiments he developed a system called *potentization*. In this system, medicines are diluted in a series of dilutions. The end result is a *non-toxic medicine* which still retains its ability to cure if it is homeopathically indicated.

This process of potentization is described in detail in *Appendix 1* at the end of the book. For a complete understanding of homeopathy, it is recommended that you read it at some point.

Suffice to say that homeopathic remedies are dispensed in different strengths referred to as *potencies*. The potency of the remedy is indicated by the number and the letter which follow the name of the medicine. For example, Pulsatilla 30C is made from the herb Pulsatilla Nigricans. It has been diluted 30 times with a dilution factor of 1/100 each time (C means centesimal). It has also been succussed (agitated by vigorous shaking) between each dilution.

The larger the number following the name of the medicine, the more times it has been diluted and shaken. Since these higher dilutions generally act longer and deeper than the lower dilutions (if well prescribed according to their homeopathic indications), they are referred to as high potencies.

This is quite different from the regular medicines with which we are all familiar, where a high potency usually means a larger dose of medicine rather than a more diluted medicine. Since they are so different, homeopathic medicines are often referred to as *remedies*. As you read on through the book, the term *remedy* will often be used when referring to these very small doses of homeopathic medicines.

Proving of medicines

For the study of substances as potential medicines, Hahnemann conducted a series of experiments called *provings*. Groups of healthy volunteers would take small doses of a substance on a daily basis. The volunteers kept journals of all symptoms they experienced in the course of the study. In this way, an accurate and consistent picture of the effects of the substance on human health could be obtained.

Hahnemann was interested in the effects of medicines on the whole person. Therefore, subjects in the provings recorded not only their physical symptoms in great detail, but also information on sleep, appetite, thirst, sensations, heat, cold, emotions, desires, thoughts, and the like.

Of special note is the fact that the medicines are proven on humans, not animals. The response of people to the substances used in provings was immediately known, even the effects on human emotions and thinking.

Anything that can cause symptoms can be studied in this way. Substances that have been studied in provings can then be used as medicines in homeopathy. In the course of homeopathic history, things as varied as herbs, minerals, poisons, foods, and bacteria have been studied and are used today as non-toxic medicines.

I got a call one day from a patient. Her daughter had been ill for a week with fever and cough. She had given her various remedies at home without success.

She said that the cough came on very bad at night when the girl lay down in bed. She had little appetite or thirst. Most peculiar was the fact that the fever came on every day at 2 PM like clockwork.

I looked in my homeopathic repertory (a book indexing symptoms with remedies) for fever at 2 PM. Sure enough, right there in black and white was her remedy, homeopathic Pulsatilla. This remedy also has cough lying down, and decreased appetite and thirst.

The patient responded dramatically to the remedy with quick resolution of her illness.

The homeopathic repertory which I consulted was written 100 years ago! Unlike much in modern medicine, the knowledge in homeopathy does not become outdated over time. On the contrary, the knowledge of the remedies and how to apply them continues to grow. Provings conducted those many years ago continue to be valid to this day.

From provings to therapy

Just as people have characteristics that distinguish them as individuals, the various provings brought out the individual nature of different medicines. Some disposed people to feel chilly, some made people warm. Some produced a thirst for large amounts of cold drinks, others for sips of warm drinks, while others caused a decreased thirst. Some caused various kinds of rashes. Some produced sensations of fear: of the dark, of dogs, of water, of death. Some produced unusual food cravings. The provings brought out the various features of each substance; what made it unique in its effects on human health.

Hahnemann then took the information from the provings and began applying it to sick patients. When a patient was found to be displaying symptoms characteristic of a particular substance, that substance was applied in small doses as a medicine.

When a proving demonstrated a symptom in the test subjects, and the substance also cured that symptom in a sick patient, that symptom was then considered a valid characteristic of that homeopathic medicine. The symptom could then be added to the compilation of medicinal indications called the homeopathic *Materia Medica.*

The Materia Medica

In homeopathy the indications for a medicine are not the disease diagnosis nor the medical condition to be treated, as is the case with conventional medicine. Instead, the homeopathic indications are simply all the various effects and symptoms which can be both caused and cured by the medicine.

In the Materia Medica, these indications are recorded for each medicine in a systematic fashion beginning with the mind and progressing throughout the different parts of the body. Indications are described in precise detail so that the practitioner can match the unique and peculiar indications for each remedy to the indications in ill patients.

Appendix 2 at the end of the book shows a remedy (in part) as a sample Materia Medica listing.

"I tried homeopathy . . . it doesn't work," the man in the back row with the raised hand said.

Curious, I asked him to explain.

"Well, homeopathy means 'like cures like,' right? So one time my daughter had the stomach flu and was throwing up a lot. I went and got her some homeopathic Ipecac. You know, the same stuff as in the medicine chest used to cause vomiting. I figured since it causes vomiting, it should work to cure it. It didn't do a thing to help."

This man still had some interest in homeopathy, or else he wouldn't be attending one of my introductory lectures.

In response I said, "This is a common mistake people make about homeopathy. You are right, 'like cures like' means that if a substance causes vomiting, it can cure vomiting. However, it must be the same type of vomiting."

"The only type of vomiting I know of is the kind where the contents of your stomach comes out," the man interjected.

"That's right, if you only look at the stomach there is just one type. But look at the whole patient. Many substances cause vomiting. Yet each one is actually different in some way. Homeopathic Ipecac works for vomiting patients if and only if they have the same symptoms which Ipecac causes. Namely, relentless nausea. This is peculiar. Most patients feel better after vomiting, but in those who need Ipecac the nausea is not relieved by vomiting.

"There are a great many possible remedies for patients with stomach flu. The appropriate remedy must be chosen for the individual for good results."

Chapter 3

The Brilliance of Homeopathy

I did my residency training at Highland Hospital in Oakland, California, a trauma center that serves a largely inner city population.

In both medical school and residency, I found it best not to advertise my naturopathic background. Some people in medicine find it interesting, but many just can't handle it. They can no longer relate to you as an intelligent or caring person, you are now one of "them."

As my training progressed, I gained much of the experience I was looking for in medicine. I became more comfortable with such things as trauma, emergencies, and intensive care.

The difference between homeopathy and conventional medicine also became more clear. Conventional medicine looks for what is the <u>same</u> between patients and then applies a uniform treatment to the disease. In homeopathy, we look for what is <u>different</u>, what makes each person unique, so we can treat the patient.

Homeopathy is simple, really. It is the whole person who is affected by disease and it is the whole person who responds to medicines.

To appreciate how the whole person is affected by disease or medicines, we have only to look at their symptoms. This is the secret to understanding how homeopathy differs from conventional medicine in a way as basic as the difference between the spherical earth and flat earth.

The disease symptoms

When someone is ill, they have many symptoms, most of which are ignored by conventional medicine but are of great importance in homeopathy. Conventional medicine recognizes and uses only those symptoms which indicate what disease the patient has.

For example, suppose a patient has asthma. They'll go to the doctor with shortness of breath and wheezing. Breathing tests will be abnormal. They may have an allergic history and often have had previous asthma attacks.

A conscientious physician may also complete a full history, exam, and laboratory evaluation. But, barring any surprises, the physician already has all the information needed to diagnose and treat the disease based on the disease symptoms. Virtually all asthmatics receive the same treatment by conventional physicians.

The signs and symptoms which were used to diagnose this disease are about the same for each person and are referred to as the *disease symptoms.* They are of little value, however, in prescribing for the whole person.

The patient's symptoms

It is the other symptoms, the ones which are either ignored or never elicited in conventional medicine, that allow a view of the whole person and the individual response to the disease.

To continue with the example of asthma, every asthmatic has many symptoms beyond the disease symptoms. The shortness of breath may be caused in one person by going into the open air, but this may relieve the shortness of breath in another. One may be thirsty for sips of cold drinks, another may have no thirst. One may be sweaty, another dry. One may feel worse after midnight, another in the morning. One may be craving salt, another sweets. One may be relieved at the seashore, another aggravated. One may be irritable, another weepy.

The point is that people respond as a whole, as an organism, to disease influences. This response is visible throughout the person as various signs and symptoms. In homeopathy, all these symptoms taken together represent the *patient's symptoms.*

It is *merely the choice* of conventional medicine to ignore the totality of the patient's symptoms because conventional medicine has no means to utilize this information. There is no need for any other than the disease symptoms when you are only treating the disease.

Medicine for the disease

Just as the disease affects the person as a whole, so do medicines. The fact that medicines affect systems throughout the body, not just in one part, is acknowledged in conventional medicine in the concept of effects and side-effects. Conventional medicines are given in large enough doses to cause a certain desired effect somewhere in the body. Other effects caused by the medicine which are not desired are termed the side-effects.

A moments reflection reveals that *there is no such thing as a medicinal side-effect.* There are only medicinal effects. The term side-effect is a euphemism for what is, in fact, an undesired effect. (It appears that the only purpose for this misleading term is to relieve the practitioner of the blame for having caused these unpleasant drug effects in the patient.)

Medicine for the patient

If you've followed the book so far, you already know that homeopathy takes a different approach and does not divide the effects of a medicine into so called effects and side-effects. Instead, the sum total of all the effects are recognized to be part of what that medicine can cause.

And, if you remember the basic principle of homeopathy ("like cures like"), the medicine can cure what it can cause. For a good response, however, the medicine must be prescribed for the patient, not the disease. This is done by matching the *patient's* symptoms (as discussed above) with the symptoms that a medicine can cause.

When a homeopathic medicine is properly prescribed, based on the similar symptoms of the whole person, it can be given in such a tiny, non-toxic dose that it will not force its effects on the body. Therefore, there are no side-effects as with drug therapy.

Treating the patient instead of the disease

This is the genius of homeopathy. It is the patient who is ill and it is the patient who responds to the medicine. *What is termed a disease by conventional medicine is merely a part of this whole* (just as the experience of the flat earth is only part of the greater reality of the round earth).

By looking at the whole patient and knowing the effects of medicines on the whole person, homeopathic practitioners are able to prescribe one **single similar medicine** for that patient. The patient's response to the medicine is then evidenced by resolution and improvement in **all the symptoms,** including those associated with the disease. The disease is cured naturally as the patient recovers.

"Dr. Dooley, it's amazing," a 40 year old woman told me on her first follow-up. "My skin rash on my hands is completely gone!"

"Skin rash?" I asked. The month before, during our initial interview, she had related all her problems to me: anxiety attacks, dry mouth, bad breath, and others; but she had said nothing about a skin rash.

"Oh, I'm so used to it and have had it all my life, that I didn't even think to mention it last month. My hands always have a dry itchy rash with cracks and fissures. But now, it's all better." She went on to explain that her other problems were also improved.

Her prescription of homeopathic Graphites would have been much easier had I known about the skin rash. But it wasn't necessary to know about it to help it. When the patient is treated as a whole, all the specific problems should improve as the patient responds.

The balance of health and disease

People who get few diseases are often referred to as healthy. In other words, the absence of disease defines their state of health. Health, however, is much more than just the absence of disease. It is more accurate to say that healthy people get fewer diseases and feel better in general because they are healthy.

This subtle distinction is important because treating disease, as is done in conventional medicine, will not necessarily result in a healthier person. It is possible for the disease to go away, and yet the patient, as a whole, remains in an equally poor, or even worse, state of health.

In such a reduced state of health, people often complain to their doctors of many symptoms such as poor energy, sleep problems, or emotional imbalance. Perhaps they just don't feel well. It is often only a matter of time before the previous disease returns or another disease, possibly more serious, takes its place.

From the flat-earth view of conventional medicine, such a new disease is then seen as an entirely different disease entity. It is treated as if there is no relationship between the old disease and the new disease. This is not so; there is a relationship.

The relationship is the patient!

These diseases do not just happen. They are processes which involve the *very same* patient.

From the homeopathic view of the whole person, the various problems and symptoms, both past and present, are all related. They reflect the unique health expression of that individual.

Furthermore, the parts of the body do not independently get sick. It is the whole person who gets sick, even though most diseases express in predominantly one part of the body or another. That is why just treating the apparently sick part may not benefit the patient as a whole.

The proof of these ideas is a cured patient, one who has been healed with a homeopathic remedy chosen for them as a whole, not just their diseases.

The short case presented above is an excellent example. If this patient had been treated in parts, the conventional way, she would have received a prescription for an anti-anxiety medicine, some cortisone lotion for her hands, and told to use breath mints or mouth wash. All of these treatments are directed at the parts, not the patient.

These treatments would have only controlled the symptoms, the outward expressions of her underlying disorder.

Using the homeopathic approach, I was able to find a remedy which matched her whole health picture. She responded as a whole and as she healed, all the problems got better, even the one I was unaware she had!

True healing, natural recovery from disease, cannot be forced. It is a process in which a person attains a higher level of health and the disease resolves naturally. This is what homeopathy is all about.

Chapter 4

A Cured Case

In the case that follows, a few minor facts have been changed to protect my patient's privacy. Otherwise, it is an accurate presentation of her, her problems, and how she was helped by homeopathy.

Initial visit : Beverly (not her real name) is a married mother of two children in her early forties. She seemed friendly and open as she related her story:

"I've had a problem with recurring cystitis (bladder infections) for many years. It mostly happens after intercourse, about one out of three times since I've been an adult.

"I've had a lot of work-up on this problem over the years. A urologic work-up shows I have two ureters on my left side. They don't think this has been causing the problem.

"If I take antibiotics right after intercourse then I have fewer infections. When I do get cystitis, it starts as a burning with urination. Then I start to feel spasms about eight to twelve hours later. It's kind of a tightening near the opening. The last drop really burns when I have to go. There is a fullness and I have to urinate frequently. If left untreated it tends to go to my left kidney.

"This problem is always in the back of my mind when I have intercourse. After the infection is treated, I have a lot of itching. Maybe that's from the antibiotics.

"I'm so tired of having it. It's more than just physical. I counseled for awhile with a teacher at the center."

Beverly paused for a moment and looked down.

"I was sexually abused as a child. He (the perpetrator) forced intercourse on me regularly from age six or seven until age twelve. After that he left the area.

"I'm going through a lot of changes right now. Spirituality is more important than it was."

She continued her story, relating some of her other problems.

"I also have a problem with my sinuses. It started when I was on vacation about seven years ago. I was pregnant then with my last child. It's a lot worse when it is wet or rainy. It's better in open air. My nose completely blocks up and I can't breath. In the morning I blow clear mucus.

"I also get a sharp pain in my left ovary area every month. It used to occur in mid-cycle, then it went away. Now it occurs just before my period."

To get a better understanding of her, I asked how her husband would describe her personality.

She replied, "He'd say I was friendly, I like people. I'm introverted and don't like to be noticed. I've always been shy; it's difficult to introduce myself. I'm honest.

"I get depressed easily. I get down on myself a lot. I have this committee in my head always pointing things out. It's like there are different personalities, like my mother saying 'do this, do that.' I've been going to counseling. It's hard to work on my sadness; there are things I'm never able to cry about.

"I get angry if someone tells me what I should be doing, if someone tells me how to feel or act or be.

"For example, the teacher at school humiliated my son. I was angry. My husband said I shouldn't feel that way. That made me even more angry."

Asked about her fears, she replied, "I'm afraid to be under a train, you know, like under an overpass. I'm afraid of being restrained, unable to move. I never felt anyone was there for me, ever. There was no one to rely on or trust. I always felt very alone. I needed to rely on myself, I needed to take care of myself.

"I dream sometimes my husband leaves and I am abandoned."

Regarding her childhood, she said, "I was introverted; I tried to be unnoticed. There was no fighting in the family. My parents did not argue. My mother was very controlling. The house was always very neat. I had a problem with anemia. Lots of times I couldn't eat. I often couldn't eat breakfast.

"My father died two years ago. We had a wonderful relationship. He never abused me. I was Daddy's little girl. He was very creative. We made doll houses, pictures. He never knew I was being abused."

She paused again in her story.

"I think about the abuse a lot. It's more of a sorrow, not an anger. I'm the only one to protect me, no one else is there. I've always felt this heavy reliance on self."

In response to specific questions, she gave the following information. She is a chilly person with cold hands and feet. Despite this, she strongly prefers to have open windows. She sleeps on her abdomen with her hands underneath her. She has warm feet and puts them out of the covers every few weeks, even in the winter.

Her period started at age 11. If she exercises regularly, she doesn't get any premenstrual symptoms. Occasionally she gets swollen breasts with some secretion.

She loves chocolate, rich creams, sauces, and ice cream. She also likes pasta, rice, potatoes and other starchy foods.

Assessment: Beverly's two medical complaints are recurring cystitis associated with intercourse, and sinus congestion. She also has a recurring left ovarian area pain with menses.

Emotionally, she carries the scars of recurring sexual abuse as a child. This issue has never been fully resolved, she often feels self-reproachful and experiences a feeling of deep sorrow. She has a persistent issue with abandonment in her life.

There were a few remedies that looked like good possibilities for Beverly. I chose to give her a remedy called Staphysagria.

Plan: Staphysagria 1M, one dose.

First follow-up (one month after initial visit)

She reported she had one episode of cystitis the first month, treated with antibiotics. She felt like she was still undergoing quite a bit of stress, "just a lot going on in my head." Her sinuses were unchanged. Her premenstrual symptoms were worse than usual that month.

Emotionally she'd been depressed, felt like giving up in life, and didn't care. She'd been more introverted, with low energy and just hadn't felt like doing much.

Assessment: Clearly, there was little, if any, response to a single dose of the remedy. I still felt this was a well indicated remedy and prescribed it again in lower potency repeated frequently.

Plan: Staphysagria 6C, one dose daily.

Second follow-up (two months after initial visit)

She had a yeast infection this past month for the first time in many years. She treated it with a topical antifungal from her gynecologist. She had cramps in her feet for one month, occasionally very severe. She once had similar cramps a few years in the past. Her period was one week early. She felt light headed for a week. She still had a lot anxiety about her life and marriage. She'd felt very busy and stressed. Her nose and sinus congestion were unchanged. She still got the left ovarian pain.

She said "I don't think the remedy is doing much. But, I've had this problem a long time and don't expect it to go away overnight."

Assessment: There was possibly some return of old symptoms (often a sign of healing), but overall no real change. Although I didn't expect her to be cured in just two months, there wasn't enough improvement to justify staying on the same remedy.

Plan: Discontinue the Staphysagria. Pulsatilla 6C, one dose daily.

Third follow-up (four months after initial visit)

This time she said she was definitely doing better. She had no episodes of cystitis. She even stopped taking the antibiotics after intercourse. Her cramps had gone away. Her stuffy nose was markedly improved. She still had some left ovarian pain the week before.

Overall, she felt emotionally much better. And her energy was improved. She said she'd been trying to communicate more with her husband and felt her relationship was improving. "It's wonderful! There has been no cystitis and this is very unusual."

She reported that she had numerous vivid dreams since she started the remedy. She dreamed of being at the ocean with her son and there were huge waves coming in. The feeling was that it was the end of the world. They ran to a tall building. Water was rising on the sides. She walked into a room with two ladies in it. They all talked about how the good times were over. Then a man came into the room and said, "Cut." It was a movie! "He said if he had told us, then he wouldn't have gotten good emotion for the film."

She said she's had these "end of the world" dreams for her entire life. "It's like there's only one hour to go, then it will all be over." She would usually wake crying, feeling that there was no one to protect her, no other adults around.

But this time was different. This dream was like a joke, "It was funny because I was so concerned, but it wasn't real."

Assessment: Excellent response to Pulsatilla.

Plan: Pulsatilla 30C, one dose weekly.

Fourth follow-up (six months after initial visit)
She did very well. It was the longest she had ever gone without a bladder infection! Her nose still got stuffy and was better if she went in the open air, but overall the stuffiness had gotten better. She had no cramps in her feet. She said her

marriage was doing better than ever. This time, her dreams were unremarkable.

Assessment: Excellent response to the remedy.

Plan: Pulsatilla 200C, one dose only.

Fifth follow-up (eight months after initial visit)

Overall, she again did well. She had no bladder infections, although she did get a few spasms that went away with cranberry juice. "This makes six months without bladder infections and that's incredible." Her marriage has been good. Emotionally, she had done well and had good energy. About the only thing that bothered her was some nose problem in the evenings.

Assessment: She is doing well, but appears to have nearly had an infection, which she kept away with cranberry juice.

Plan: Pulsatilla 1M, one dose only.

Sixth follow-up (ten months after initial visit)

Doing fine. No problems. No cystitis. Nose much better, occasional slight stuffiness. Feeling emotionally good, no big highs and lows. Feels more "up." Doing volunteer work at spiritual center.

Assessment: Doing great!

Plan: Wait. No medication needed. Follow-up as needed.

This is the kind of case we love in homeopathy. Once the right remedy was prescribed, her recurring problem of about twenty years duration was gone.

Not only did her main complaint get better, but, as we'll discuss in more detail, she improved dramatically on all levels. She experienced increased energy, a greater sense of well being, and resolution or improvement in all complaints. This type of response is characteristic in homeopathy and demonstrates what happens when the whole person is treated instead of just the disease.

The remedy which cured her, Pulsatilla, is in *no way* a specific medicine for recurring cystitis. It was NOT prescribed for her cystitis. *It was prescribed for her as a person.* Her characteristics that strongly indicated this remedy include such things as her mild nature, her timidity, her tendency to be a pleaser, her lifelong sense of abandonment, her amelioration in open air, her chilliness coupled with a desire for open air, her hot feet in bed, and her food desires.

Staphysagria is also a common remedy in patients with recurring cystitis, especially associated with intercourse. Staphysagria is also a frequently indicated remedy in patients with such a history of sexual abuse. Patients needing either remedy can appear very mild and yielding. Although Staphysagria appeared to be a good prescription, she received no benefit from it.

The conventional approach in this case was incapable of curing her tendency to these infections over the years. Despite sophisticated urologic work-ups, there was nothing to help her other than taking antibiotics for each episode and after intercourse.

Beverly possibly needed this remedy her whole life. It appears if she had taken the Pulsatilla many years earlier, she could have avoided the ten to twelve bladder infections per year, expensive work-ups, and repeated antibiotic use.

An important aspect of this case was the unresolved emotional trauma resulting from her sexual abuse as a child. The allopathic care she received did nothing to address this issue. Whereas the counseling she received helped to some extent, it was only after receiving the *simillimum* (curative similar remedy) did she experience a sense of emotional well being and a lifting of the "deep sorrow."

This is a common experience in homeopathy. A homeopathic remedy cannot substitute for human compassion and understanding, yet it is common for patients to finally reach a stage of resolution and attain an ability to move ahead in life after a good prescription. This is because emotions are closely related to a person's glands and nerves. As these glands and nerves heal, the associated emotional qualities are strengthened and expressed in a more balanced way.

Beverly experienced some of this process in her dreams. Under the action of the remedy her dream state became very vivid. She experienced many of the recurring emotional issues in these dreams during this period. As the healing progressed, she felt a resolution in the dream state which corresponded with a similar resolution and feeling of emotional well being in her day-to-day life.

Homeopaths find this to be true: *a person's experience in emotional and mental life cannot be separated from their physical complaints.* It is the patient who is ill, and this illness is simply expressed or reflected in many ways.

This is why homeopathy can often help patients even when the disease diagnosis is unclear or unknown. All the various symptoms and signs of the patient — including physical, mental, and emotional — are used as guideposts for understanding the expression of the person's health-maintaining mechanism. The appropriate remedy stimulates this mechanism and a healing response occurs.

This case also shows the use of the two systems of dosing, the daily dose and the single dose. These are described in more detail in *Chapter 8*. It should also be noted how the potencies given to Beverly gradually ascended as she responded. As her health and vitality increased she was able to respond to the increasingly subtle doses of remedy in a gentle and permanent manner.

Finally notice how the wisdom of the body heals the more important organs first. Her stuffy nose — not a serious problem — was her only remaining complaint after many months of treatment. Even this minor complaint became progressively better as healing continued.

Beverly had realistic expectations of how fast homeopathy could help her. Even though results were negligible after the first few months, she felt her problems were of a longstanding nature and would take some time to resolve.

Beverly got results with homeopathy largely because she was open and candid with personal aspects of her life and history. The things which people are most hesitant to discuss or examine often contain the clues for cure in homeopathy. These clues reflect pathology on an inner level. Healing the person, as opposed to the disease, may be difficult without such an understanding.

Chapter 5

A Brief History

A Victorian era joke about homeopathy:
    A well dressed woman entered a homeopathic pharmacy.
    "Sir," she enquired of the pharmacist. "I would like to purchase one four-hundredth of a grain of phosphate of magnesia, please."
    "I'm sorry, madam," the pharmacist replied coolly. "We do not sell in quantities that large."

Homeopathy in the ancient world

Samuel Hahnemann did not discover homeopathy. The basic concept of homeopathy, being the therapeutic action of similars, has been discovered many times throughout human history. It was mentioned and used by Hippocrates and a variety of practices based on homeopathic principles have come and gone over time.

One such practice used in ancient India was called *visa chikitsa*. It was developed approximately 3,500 years ago in the era now referred to as the Mahabharata age. This visa chikitsa is discussed in the book *Discourses on Mahabharata* by P.R. Sarkar, in the chapter entitled "Medical Science of the Age." (English edition 1981, Ananda Press, Calcutta, India)

In this system, various types of poisonous venoms were applied to treat the bites of poisonous animals. For example, snake venom, spider venom, and scorpion venom were used to treat snake bite, spider bite, and scorpion bite.

In one of the stories from this Mahabharata era, a character named Bhiima was poisoned by his enemies, the Kaoravas. The experts in ayurveda (traditional Indian medicine) then gave injections of poison to Bhiima and he was cured. This shows the people of that era were familiar with the principle of using poisons to treat poisons.

Homeopathy, as developed by Hahnemann, does not use injections. The medicines are absorbed simply by coming in contact with a mucous membrane surface, such as under the tongue.

The visa chikitsa system of using poisons to treat poisonings was neglected over the course of time and is no longer in use.

The science of homeopathy

Although Dr. Hahnemann did not discover homeopathy, he deserves full credit for developing homeopathy into a science. His observations, insights, method, and application stand today as a scientific achievement rarely, if ever, paralleled.

Before the time of Hahnemann, homeopathy existed only in rudimentary form. There was no well developed system for discovering medicines or for applying them to patients. Cures did happen, but they were often based more on empiricism or luck. The observation of similars had been made, but no one had realized its potential or implications.

Medicine in the time of Hahnemann

The conventional system of medicine in which Hahnemann trained can only be described as crude. Popular theories came and went as to the supposed cause of disease. Treatments likewise changed regularly over time.

The treatments of the day were often dramatic, brutal, or dangerous — large doses of toxic minerals like mercury were common. Purgatives were given in large doses to evacuate the bowels. Sudorifics were given to induce sweating. Intentionally bleeding a patient was a common practice — patients were relieved of blood until their ears rang (a sign of impending shock) and they were pale from acute blood loss. At that point the bleeding was stopped, as no more "bad humors" could be expelled without endangering the patient's life.

Physicians at that time were considered well-educated. They had studied their art in large prestigious institutions. They kept up with the latest advances in the medical sciences such as physiology, pathology, and anatomy. People today look back and gasp at the fundamental ignorance of these practitioners. "How is it," people query, "that these physicians could overlook the most basic and common sense elements of biologic processes and life? How could they think these brutal treatments could benefit anyone?"

At the time these treatments were popular, they actually correlated with the level of disease perception. The fact is: *no disease-oriented treatment can be effective beyond the perception of the disease.*

For example, fever was perceived as an over-abundance of blood — you could see the red face and feel the bounding pulse. After bleeding the patient, the red face would be gone and the pulse less bounding. These findings tended to confirm the erroneous perception and treatment of fever in the minds of both the physician and populace. Today, disease-oriented treatments sometimes suffer from this same shortsightedness.

Physicians of that era were exclusively male. They maintained a tight society and exerted their influence against those perceived as crossing into their territory.

The true healers of the era, before the advent of homeopathy, were the herbalists. Mostly female, they practiced an art passed through the generations that respected the fundamental ability of the body to heal itself. The patient of that era was fortunate to be in the hands of such a healer. With nutritious broths and simple herbal medicines, the patient's chances of recovery were actually enhanced by the treatment.

These herbalists were largely opposed by the medical establishment. They were belittled as backwards, uneducated, or even dangerous. Many women persecuted as witches were actually herbal healers, performing their services, often without remuneration, for the welfare of the community.

Such was the medical world in which Hahnemann trained. Being a man of integrity as well as profound intelligence, he discontinued this practice of medicine which he perceived as harmful.

Hahnemann starts a revolution

Hahnemann went on to support himself by translating medical texts, new and old, in and out of his native German language. In the course of this translating work he was exposed to the idea of similars. He performed his first experiments on himself, taking daily doses of Cinchona (quinine) until he developed symptoms similar to malaria (which Cinchona was used to treat).

Little did Hahnemann know when he conducted this first experiment with Cinchona that it was the start of a revolution in healthcare. Within his own lifetime, this change in thinking would result in a bitter schism in the world of medicine.

Homeopathy was nothing short of revolutionary. It brought together a new level of scientific method and objectivity with a profound respect for the inherent ability of the organism to heal itself. It depended not on changing theories and discoveries, but on the observation that each individual manifests illness in an individual way. It utilized this observation in a system that brought unparalleled results.

As word of Hahnemann's accomplishments spread, students and physicians from all over Europe came to study and work with him, thereby further expanding the frontiers of this new science.

Organized medicine opposes homeopathy

Acceptance was far from universal. Despite the irrefutable success of homeopathy, not only in acute epidemic diseases such as typhoid and cholera, but also in chronic disease, the medical community as a whole did not embrace homeopathy.

There were various reasons for this rejection. One was Hahnemann himself. As he refined this new therapeutic science, he saw more clearly than ever the terrible effects of allopathic medicine on health. He became an outspoken critic of allopathy, denouncing its barbaric and irrational methodologies in the strongest terms. Physicians of the "old school" felt threatened by these attacks and tended to ban together to defend their position. In the early years, every physician practicing homeopathy was a convert from allopathy and physicians were compelled to take a stand on one side or the other of this issue.

Many allopathic physicians felt homeopathy was just too different. For one thing, it was more difficult to practice. There was no single treatment for a given diagnosis, each patient had to be studied individually. To take up the practice, a physician had to retrain in an entirely new system (this is still true today). Physicians were accustomed to forcing the system with large dramatic doses of poisons and the homeopathic doses seemed to be too small. It was inconceivable to them that these non-toxic infinitesimal doses were capable of eliciting a response.

Homeopathy crosses the Atlantic

Despite the opposition, homeopathy moved ahead. At the time of Hahnemann's death in 1843, homeopathy was well known throughout Europe and America. About 100 medicines had been well-proven and their therapeutic effectiveness established.

Homeopathy came to America in the 1820s. Here, as in Europe, homeopathy became a divisive issue in the medical community. Emotions often ran high, with medical society meetings sometimes degenerating into shouting matches between the opposing camps.

The homeopaths formed the first national medical association, the American Institute of Homeopathy (AIH), in 1844. This association exists to this day representing medical doctors who practice homeopathy.

The allopaths were not to be outdone. They countered by forming the American Medical Association (AMA) in 1846. Letters between the founding members of the AMA show that one of the main purposes for the formation of the AMA was to oppose the spread and practice of homeopathy. Early AMA members also opposed the spread of osteopathy (a medical system using manipulation of the joints and other tissues).

This contentious relationship continued throughout the 1800s. Homeopathy continued to spread and homeopathic medical schools were started. Despite the often desperate and unprofessional attempts by the AMA to discredit and stop homeopathy, *by the turn of the century one in four physicians in America was a homeopath.*

There were homeopathic hospitals, homeopathic medical schools, homeopathic medical journals, homeopathic societies, homeopathic manufacturers, and homeopathic pharmacies. The discerning observer in contemporary museums will see that the medical kits of the nineteenth century physicians on display often contain homeopathic medicines.

Homeopathy was extremely popular, especially among the intelligentsia and aristocracy. To this day, the personal physician of the Queen of England is a homeopath. Homeopathy went with the British to India where it sank deep roots. The oldest continuously operating medical college in Asia is the homeopathic medical school in Calcutta. It still teaches homeopathy.

The twentieth century

With the advent of the twentieth century came a sharp change in the momentum of homeopathy, especially in America. There was no single reason for this decline, nor did homeopathy suddenly became ineffective. A combination of changing social, political, scientific, and economic trends conspired to make homeopathy a nearly forgotten footnote of American medical history in just one generation.

One such trend was the application of scientific advances in allopathic medicine. Disease diagnosis improved and allopathic therapies began to reflect rationality in their approach. Antibiotics cured many diseases which before had been difficult to treat. New medical and surgical techniques captured the imagination of a society infatuated with science and scientific progress.

The Flexner report of 1906 resulted in tighter regulation of medical school curricula and standards. Homeopathic medical schools were faced with the adoption of allopathic curricula and pharmaceutical labs or with the loss of accreditation and funding. Over time, the remaining homeopathic courses in these schools were abandoned. The average MD graduate today of Hahnemann Medical College in Philadelphia is ignorant not only of homeopathic theory and practice, but also of their own school's history.

Joining the ranks of a waning homeopathic profession held little attraction to the youth of the early 1900s. Fewer and fewer joined the profession and the existing vanguard gradually grew old and died.

Survival into the 1960s

By the 1960s there remained only a relative handful of competent homeopathic practitioners in the United States. There were no homeopathic medical schools, no homeopathic hospitals, and few homeopathic pharmacies. The American Institute of Homeopathy survived, but those wishing to learn homeopathy had to undertake an apprenticeship with an accomplished practitioner or go overseas to study. National College of Naturopathic Medicine was perhaps the only professional institution in the country which taught homeopathy as part of its regular curricula.

Throughout the rest of the world homeopathy survived in better shape. The Royal London Homeopathic Hospital continued its operation. Homeopathy continued in France and Germany, though with a smaller percentage of practitioners. Homeopathy actually grew in India, where the low cost of homeopathic medicines and non-reliance on expensive technology encouraged its practice.

Homeopathic revival

Since the 1970s, awareness of and interest in homeopathy has steadily increased. Patients frustrated with the limitations, side-effects, and high costs of conventional medicine actively seek health-oriented alternatives.

Homeopathy is a logical choice. It can be used in patients with both acute and chronic conditions, has few, if any, side-effects, and is inexpensive.

In America, the homeopaths of the past were almost all medical doctors. Today, medical doctors practicing homeopathy represent a minority of the practitioners. Many practitioners hold licenses as naturopaths, chiropractors, nurse practitioners, physician assistants, and acupuncturists. There are also a growing number of professional homeopaths, persons with no formal medical training or licensing outside of their homeopathic training. Some of the most renowned homeopaths in the world today fall in this category.

Professional associations and certification

A number of associations now certify homeopathic competence in different professions. Professional homeopaths in Europe may register with the Society of Homeopaths. The North American Society of Homeopaths represents professional homeopaths on this side of the Atlantic. The American Institute of Homeopathy certifies medical doctors. State homeopathic medical boards regulate medical doctors practicing homeopathy in Nevada and Arizona. The Homeopathic Academy of Naturopathic Physicians certifies naturopaths.

There has been a movement in recent years for the development of a single exam and certification for all practitioners. What was once a profession by and for medical doctors is gradually becoming an independent profession.

Chapter 6

Non-toxic Medicines

A patient's experience

A 48 year old woman returned for her first follow-up. Her phone report three weeks earlier had been positive; she was sleeping better and experiencing less anxiety. Her remedy was homeopathic arsenic (Arsenicum Album), 9C potency, one dose daily. She began her report:

"First of all, I have to tell you what happened. Two weeks ago I had my once yearly check-up with my gynecologist. She has a form where the patient is supposed to fill out new things. So I mentioned, perhaps it was a mistake, about what I'm doing here. You can guess what happened! I told her I was seeing a homeopath and was taking very small doses of arsenic. The woman turned bright red! As red as that carpet! She had a conniption FIT! She said, 'I can't believe you'd take something like that!' She told me that arsenic in any dose is a poison, that it is toxic to the liver, and that the liver does not regenerate. She warned me to stop taking it IMMEDIATELY! She said it was the craziest thing she'd ever heard of. She demanded, DEMANDED, that I not take this anymore.

"When I got home my husband asked, 'Did you tell her you're going to a homeopath?' I told him what she said and he absolutely insisted that I not take anymore Arsenicum until I talk with you. So I haven't taken any for the last 2 weeks."

Perhaps this gynecologist was acting in what she felt was the best interest of her patient. Unfortunately, her good intentions reflected an appalling and inexcusable ignorance.

The fact is, there exists no prescription medicine that this gynecologist can prescribe which is as non-toxic as the remedy she censured. None. Nor does there exist another over-the-counter medicine which is as harmless and safe as this 9C potency homeopathic remedy. None.

It is the unimaginable smallness of the dose which assures the non-toxicity of homeopathic remedies. It is the great discovery of homeopathy that these micro-doses of substances, if prepared according to the serial dilution method introduced by Hahnemann, retain their ability to stimulate a response in the organism when, and only when, homeopathically indicated.

To better understand some of this chapter, you need to remember that homeopathic remedies are prepared through a series of dilutions. The higher the number, the more times it has been diluted. It is recommended you read *Appendix 1* (at the end of the book) where this process is described in more detail.

Meta-molecular medicines

To give some idea how small these doses are, consider a concept of chemistry known as Avogadro's number. This extremely large number (about 602,000,000,000,000,000, 000,000) represents the number of particles (atoms or molecules) present in a given volume of a substance (a gram mole). Simply stated, when this number is surpassed in the process of dilution, there will statistically remain no atoms or molecules of the original substance left. This occurs at approximately the 12 C (or 24 X) potency.

In other words, potencies higher than the 12 C (or 24 X) have no molecules of the original substance remaining. Yet homeopaths routinely use potencies vastly higher than these with great success. Therefore, some property of the original substance must be transferred to the diluent (diluting liquid) in the process of serial dilutions.

To this day, the nature of this transferred property or how a patient responds to it is not well understood. However, many observations have been made about homeopathic remedies that can help to clarify their nature and action.

Proper preparation is essential

The dilutions used in preparing remedies must be properly agitated between each dilution step. Failure to do so results in loss of the remedy's ability to stimulate a homeopathic response in the patient. Hence, agitation is clearly a necessary part of the process in which the homeopathic properties of the original substance are transferred to the diluting liquid.

Immunity to oxidation

Most medicines and vitamins, if left open to the air, will spoil. The oxygen in the air reacts with the molecules of the medicine and causes them to degrade. This process is called oxidation. Homeopathic remedies, however, do not spoil in this way. This is consistent with the notion that there is some non-molecular property of the remedy which causes a response in the patient.

Sensitivity to electromagnetic properties

Remedies are not damaged by the oxygen in the air, but they are sensitive to electromagnetic fields. They can easily be damaged by exposure to such things as direct sunlight, microwave, high external heat, large magnetic fields, and the like.

This suggests that some kind of electromagnetic pattern (or another similar energetic property) is transferred to the diluting liquid during the dilution process.

Mechanism of action not understood

The exact nature of this energetic property or how a living organism responds to it is not understood. Various theories have been proposed and research into these areas is ongoing.

The fact that the mechanism of action of homeopathic remedies has not been well defined does not change in any way their usefulness or effectiveness. It is common that understanding why something works is discovered long after it has been in use.

For example, sailors ate fresh fruits to cure the disease known as scurvy hundreds of years before it was understood that a substance called vitamin C in the fruit is what the body needed. In conventional medicine today, the mechanism of action of many, if not most, medicines is poorly understood. The mechanism of action of common aspirin was not understood even partially until recent decades.

Homeopathy violates no known laws of chemistry, biology, or physics. Such a notion, sometimes promoted by skeptics of homeopathy, is ridiculous. Homeopathy was and is a therapeutic science based on objectively reproducible data and clinical experience.

There is always a tendency in science to reject new observations based on their apparent disagreement with the accepted view. This kind of thinking is what is referred to in this book as flat-earth. Such a mediocre mentality was and is a main stumbling block to scientific progress.

"The poison control center said it has toxic alkaloids," he said.

"I know, but the dose was too small for any danger of toxicity," I replied.

"But he ate the WHOLE bottle!" he exclaimed.

So what do I say to an emergency physician who just unnecessarily pumped a child's stomach?

I was still practicing as a naturopath in southern Oregon at the time. The patient with the breast infection at the beginning of Chapter 1, called me to report her three-year-old son had eaten a bottle of homeopathic Pulsatilla 30C. He "had to get his stomach pumped out" but was doing fine. Why she hadn't called me first I couldn't fathom. I thought I should call the doctor to let him know, for future reference, that these medicines are non-toxic.

If you've followed the book so far, and read Appendix 1, you'll appreciate my dilemma.

Here is a conventional physician, getting a call from a naturopath claiming that the poison control center was right, Pulsatilla is toxic, but then again, this Pulsatilla wasn't.

Should I say the dose is so small there are no molecules? Then why did I prescribe it? How can a medicine do something if it doesn't exist?

How can I explain homeopathy in a few sentences under such circumstances?

The answer is, I can't. This physician had no background nor interest in understanding or even discussing these kinds of ideas.

So, in the end, all I could say was, "It was a very small dose, less than part of one drop in the whole bottle. The toxic dose is much higher than that."

"Oh," he replied.

A biologic principle

Homeopaths today accept homeopathy as a fundamental principle. That is, living things can respond to properly prepared and homeopathically indicated microdilutions of substances. As a fundamental principle, homeopathy is not subject to failure.

To clarify, consider the example of aerodynamics. If an airplane crashes no one says that the laws of aerodynamics have failed or are invalid. People have instead failed in the application of the laws. In the same way, if a patient does not benefit from homeopathic treatment, it does not mean the principle of homeopathy has failed or is invalid. It is the people who have failed in its application.

Hahnemann's perspective

Samuel Hahnemann was an accomplished chemist and was aware of the fact that homeopathic dilutions went beyond the commonly understood material realm. Yet, as a scientist, he could not deny the objective validity of his observations. He observed that the reaction of patients to homeopathic remedies was a process involving the whole person and so relied on a concept known as vital force, which is discussed in the next chapter.

Chapter 7

Understanding Vital Force

Have you ever bought a bag of oranges only to find that one orange in the middle of the bag is rotten? It is mushy and covered with fungus.

Surprisingly, the neighboring oranges are often fine, despite the fact they are in direct contact with the fungus. You just rinse them off and they are quite edible.

The point is that the fungus does not, by itself, cause the oranges to rot. They must first be susceptible to fungal attack, which happens when they have lost vitality through aging or damage. In this degenerate state, the fungus can take hold.

In a similar way, people can only contract diseases when they are susceptible to them. By addressing this susceptibility, homeopathic treatment allows for natural resolution of disease.

An old and well-known concept

In the era prior to modern science, various concepts of vital force were widely accepted. This is an invisible, immaterial, yet dynamic force which animates the physical body. This vital principle maintains all the parts of the material body, both sensation and function, in a harmonious and coordinated manner. The mind and will can then express higher purpose in life. Without this vital force, the material body is incapable of any sensation or function; in other words, is dead.

Ideas similar to vital force are still in use today. In oriental medicine and martial arts this force is referred to as *chi*, meaning life-force. In yoga and ayurveda it is called *prana*, meaning vital energy.

Hahnemann on vital force

In his book, *Organon of Medicine*, Hahnemann discusses the basic theories and practice of homeopathy. Hahnemann proposed that the essence of illness is a disorder in the vital force. Because of this disorder, people are susceptible to various diseases and afflictions. When the integrity of the vital force is restored, the whole organism recovers health and the disease is cured.

Other natural forces are invisible. Gravity and magnetism cannot be seen but are inferred by their effects. Hahnemann felt that the effects of a single disorder in the vital force results in many signs and symptoms throughout the patient. By viewing the totality of the patient's signs and symptoms, a picture of the disturbance on the vital force can emerge, even though the vital force itself cannot be directly examined.

Hahnemann also felt that homeopathic remedies are sufficiently subtle to directly correct morbid derangements in the vital force.

In short, this was part of his theory explaining the observation that a single homeopathic remedy can result in improved health and the resolution of symptoms throughout the patient.

Rejected by modern science

Modern science currently teaches that vital force is an outdated and discredited theory. It is now generally accepted that all of these life functions are the result of biochemical processes. These processes utilize the same basic elements and chemical properties inside living things as occur outside of living things. Therefore, it is felt that there is no need for any force which is unique to life.

Homeopathic practitioners are conversant with the tenets of modern science. They have studied biochemistry and other sciences which explain the chemical basis of life processes. Yet homeopaths today still utilize the term vital force in describing both the patient and the effects of medicines on the patient. In doing so, homeopaths do not reject the well established concepts of science. The problem is a matter of terminology and perspective.

The whole person view

Looking at and evaluating the whole person is entirely different from looking at and evaluating the sum of the parts. Science and medicine today are concerned almost exclusively with the parts. Disease research attempts to understand the problem on the most refined biochemical level available. Treatment is likewise directed at this level.

Vital force, however, is a concept of the whole, living person and has little relevance in scientific studies which investigate only the parts of an organism. It has been lost sight of in conventional medicine and contemporary science. Homeopathy is the therapeutic science of the whole person. It needs concepts and terms which allow the perception and evaluation of the person in a unified way. Vital force remains the most appropriate and useful term for this purpose.

A unifying factor

It is not necessary that one must be a believer in vital force or a convert to vitalism to practice homeopathy or to benefit from its application as a patient. Those who do practice homeopathy, however, come to appreciate patients in progressively subtler ways and eventually perceive a great unity of human life.

A unifying factor becomes evident in all the aspects of life, from the very mundane, such as a dry patch on the elbow, to the subtle expressions of the mind, such as spiritual aspiration.

This unifying factor — the vital force — represents a whole which is synergistically greater than the sum of the parts. Perhaps vital force is an invisible bioenergetic force which cannot yet be independently measured but whose effects can be observed in living beings. Or, as skeptics feel, perhaps it is just an appearance, a kind of illusion, caused by the sum of the known and unknown biochemical processes of the body.

In one sense, it doesn't matter. Neither possibility changes the reality or practice of homeopathy. Vital force continues to be a useful model for perceiving disease influences and medicinal effects on the whole person.

Chapter 8

Healing with Homeopathy

"The remedy didn't work," he stated bluntly at his first follow-up.

"I'm sorry to hear that," I replied. "How is your problem doing?"

"It's not bothering me anymore, it went away."

"If it went away, why do you say the remedy didn't work?"

"Well, it seems like it just got well on its own, that's all."

I've had this same conversation a number of times over the years. No one can say for sure if the remedy helped this particular man, or if he "just got well" coincidentally. But that is exactly what happens when you heal naturally, you "just get well."

The following questions and answers about homeopathic healing concern patients with health problems of a chronic nature, that is, problems of long duration or frequent recurrence.

How long will it take before I notice a change?

Most patients with a chronic health problem notice a change in about one to four weeks.

What will I notice first?

The first change is often improved energy and disposition. Since natural healing occurs from the inside out, a sense of well-being, improved sleep, and other energy changes usually occur before the physical changes.

Sometimes the initial changes are subtle — those around you may recognize them before you do yourself.

Occasionally, there is an increased need for sleep in the initial stages of healing. It is as if you need more down time for repairs. This is a good sign.

How long until I'm well?

That depends. If you've been sick a long time with stubborn problems, it may take a number of years before you're fully healed. Some people, like Beverly whose case is presented in *Chapter 4,* respond with remarkable quickness despite the fact they've had their problems a long time.

Then how will I know if I'm getting better?

You will feel better and your problems will be resolving.

Homeopaths usually see patients every four to eight weeks or so. The idea is to be able to stand back and see the forest instead of the trees. In other words, to be able to see the changes and improvement in the whole person over time and not just the day-to-day changes. There should be overall improvement week-to-week and month-to-month.

This improvement, however, is rarely uninterrupted. Most people take three steps ahead and then one back as they heal. That's why it's necessary to stand back to interpret the changes.

Why did my friend get worse before she got better?

Sometimes healing is a bit like cleaning house — it's a little messier when you're in the middle of cleaning than before you started.

But even when that happens, you usually feel better anyway. Your energy is better and you have a sense of well-being in spite of the fact that some of your symptoms may be temporarily increased as your body cleans house.

This response is sometimes called an *aggravation.*

How often should I take the remedy?

The practitioner will tell you how to take it.

There are two main ways remedies are given. Either as a single dose given one time only (usually a high potency) or as a daily dose repeated over time (usually a lower potency). Both of these systems were used by Hahnemann himself in one form or another.

Choosing one method over the other depends on the patient, their problems, other medications they may be on, their age, and other factors.

The goal is a gentle and permanent cure.

If I'm getting better, why should I follow-up?

As you heal, your response to the remedy will tend to fade eventually at a given potency. It is necessary to gradually increase the potency of the remedy until the healing is permanent.

Knowing when to increase the potency and by how much takes training and experience. Repeating remedies too soon or in the wrong potency can sometimes delay or disrupt healing.

If you just keep taking a remedy without change, it is possible to get a proving of that medicine, that is, the medicine will start to give you symptoms. This is not dangerous — simply discontinuing the remedy will stop the process. It is another reason, however, why follow-up is important.

Will I need more than one remedy?

Sometimes. A practitioner will rarely change remedies, though, until you have stopped responding to the remedy you are on.

It may take more than one remedy before a good healing response begins. Over the course of time, some people need new remedies as they are affected by new circumstances of life and as their improved health presents a new symptom picture.

What will get well first?

Different problems often do not heal simultaneously. The more "inner" and serious problems tend to heal first, the more "outer" and less serious problems may follow. This is just the way the body's wisdom works.

It may turn out that your body's priorities are different than yours in what should heal first. What you consider to be the main problem may be one of the last things your body heals.

For example, you may be concerned about your acne for cosmetic reasons, but to your body, this is a minor problem that is superficial. As you respond to a remedy, your sleep may improve, your anxiety be relieved, and your digestive problems corrected before the skin fully clears.

In a situation like this, you must trust your body and allow it to heal in its own way. This aspect of healing cannot be forced. Homeopathy works with the natural recuperative processes of the body but does not control them.

What does return of old symptoms mean?

It means that less serious problems which you've had in the past sometimes return as you heal. This is usually an excellent sign. What appears to happen is that as you heal, you reach a higher level of health. When you regain the same level of health as in the past, you re-experience the health problems which you had at that time. Concurrent with this, the more serious problems for which you are being treated should resolve. As you continue to heal, the returning problems will also resolve.

For example, it's not uncommon during a follow-up for a patient to make a comment such as, "It's strange. My nervous condition is much better, but a rash I haven't had in years in bothering me. What should I do about it?"

The answer is, "*Nothing!* Let it heal from the inside out, and then both the rash and the nervous condition will be gone. Treating the rash topically may cause it to be suppressed. In such *disease suppression*, the rash might go away, but the nervous condition would return."

What about acute diseases?

Acute diseases are the more short term kinds of illnesses. Examples are colds, flu, diarrhea, ear infections, and the like. (The first case presented in the book of the woman with a breast infection is an example of an acute illness.)

The information above for chronic illnesses has little application in acute conditions. In acute cases, remedies are given in a wide range of potencies and with a variety of dosing schedules.

Results are expected in minutes to days, depending on the patient and the condition. Remedies may be changed frequently or repeated often depending on the needs of the patient.

Some of the self-care books which describe this process in more detail are referenced in *Appendix 3*. You should understand that homeopathy can be very effective in acute diseases, but remember that the same principle of treating the patient, instead of the disease, still applies.

Chapter 9

How to Get Results

A patient with chronic fatigue syndrome was doing remarkably better at her one month follow-up, in fact, better than she had done in the past one and a half years. She had no more low grade fevers, no headaches, was sleeping better, needed less sleep, and had energy to live her life. She was delighted and looking forward to continued improvement. She was scheduled for another appointment in two months and told to call if there was any problem. She was told to continue to observe the do's and don'ts previously recommended, as she was still responding to the remedy.

Five weeks later I received a call from her. "Dr. Dooley," she lamented. "I was feeling so good I decided it wouldn't hurt if I drank just one cup of coffee. That was just two days ago. Now I feel as bad as I did before I came to see you. What should I do?"

We repeated the remedy and she again responded well, but it took some time before she regained the same level of wellness she had experienced before the coffee. Coffee does not cause such a reaction in all patients, but clearly this patient needs to strictly avoid it during this period of recovery.

Classical homeopathy

Homeopathy refers to the science of prescribing medicines for the patient (as opposed to the disease) according to the similar symptoms. The medicines are prescribed in minute homeopathic doses because these small doses are safe and effective. But it is not the smallness of the dose nor the way it is prepared that makes it homeopathic. It is homeopathic when the basis of the prescription is the similarity of symptoms between the remedy and the patient.

Since early in the history of homeopathy people have repeatedly developed different methods for prescribing homeopathic remedies. These methods are based on pathological diagnosis, body types, colonic flora, personality, acupuncture points, and others. Most of these were developed in an attempt to make homeopathy easier.

To distinguish themselves from these other systems, many practitioners use the term *classical homeopathy* to refer to the original homeopathic system of prescribing for the patient as a whole based on the similar symptoms.

The information in this chapter about how to get good results with homeopathy applies to the system of classical homeopathy (which we have discussed throughout this book).

The practitioner

Good results with homeopathy depend largely on the skill of the practitioner in perceiving the patient and prescribing a remedy which will cause a good homeopathic response in the patient. There is a lot that the patient can do, however, to enhance or detract from their chances of a good prescription and response.

Be committed

Homeopathy is new and different for the average patient. Some approach it with skepticism and figure they'll try it and see what happens. These patients often quit before good results are achieved.

The best way to get results is to make homeopathy your primary form of therapy. That is to say, homeopathy is what you think of first and pursue first in your healthcare needs. As a medical doctor, I say with conviction that conventional medicine is what should be used secondarily, as a backup to homeopathy, and not the other way around. A patient should first give their system a chance to heal naturally and only resort to drug therapy when truly necessary.

Many practitioners have one or two older patients who were raised on homeopathy, where homeopathy was the primary therapy for the family throughout their lives. These patients are different. They are easier to prescribe for and their systems respond well to the remedies.

Most patients of conventional medicine tend to have been over-medicated throughout their lives. Their systems have been constantly forced with large doses of drugs and rarely given a chance to heal naturally. As a result, the expression of their health-maintaining mechanism is often blunted and confused. Over time, under homeopathic care, this situation tends to resolve itself and their systems start to work in a manner more like those patients who have had primary homeopathic care for many years.

Patients with chronic health problems who are just starting with homeopathy should realize it may take a number of years for full recovery from these problems. Chronic health problems do not appear overnight. Often, patients suffer for years before the identifiable problems surface. It is unrealistic to think these problems will just evaporate after a few months of homeopathic care.

Unfortunately many people do just that. They constantly jump from one form of therapy to another, never allowing their problems to heal. As the years go by, they merely chase symptoms throughout their body while their health gradually deteriorates.

Patients who want results with homeopathy, or any form of therapy for that matter, need to be committed. This means following the advice of the practitioner, scheduling follow-up appointments as directed, and working with the practitioner when problems arise.

Prepare for the interview

The main tool used in homeopathy for evaluating patients is the interview. Good results in homeopathy depend on how well the practitioner can understand you and your problems.

There are a huge number of popular psychological books and media shows today. As a result, many people express their problems and feelings in terms of a therapist's diagnosis instead of just simply stating their experience.

For example, the statement, "I'm co-dependent due to my dysfunctional family upbringing," means many different things depending on who says it. The patient may mean they are unassertive, timid, and avoid conflict. They may suffer from anxieties and worry. Perhaps they were abused in some manner as a child or are currently in an abusive relationship. They may be abusive. They may burst into tears at the drop of a hat or fly easily into rages. They may be self-reproachful, have suicidal thoughts or other problems.

Stress is another experience in life that is very individual. A given stressful situation will cause stress in fifty individuals for fifty different reasons. Stress is actually subjective — it depends entirely on the make-up of that individual. For this reason, homeopaths usually prefer to hear examples of your stress and how you reacted, not just that you are undergoing stress.

This same principle of stating your experience also holds true for the medical diagnoses as well. A strep throat is experienced in different ways by different people. Some are better by cold drinks, some by warm, some by swallowing solid food. Some patients want their neck covered, others open. In some the pain is worse in the evenings, others in the morning.

Please write down things you want to discuss ahead of time so you won't forget. Of importance to homeopaths are the things we can't see about you, the things you must tell us.

The best advice is to just be yourself. Don't try and say what you think a doctor wants to hear. Just tell your story as you would to a close friend.

One night I was eating dinner with my oldest son, Eamon. He was three years old at the time. Suddenly he held up his three-pronged fork and stared at it. "Dad!" he exclaimed. "This isn't a fork, it's a threek!"

From his perspective, he was absolutely right. None the less, I went on to explain that the word fork is not derived from the word four and that a fork can have any number of prongs. He listened somewhat skeptically while regarding the "threek" he still held in his hand. In the end he just smiled and kept on eating.

Even common words mean different things to different people. Don't be surprised if your practitioner asks to hear examples of what you are saying in order to better understand you as an individual.

Interviewing the family

Throughout the history of homeopathy, interviewing other family members to get a better understanding of the patient has been practiced. For young children, a correct prescription usually depends primarily on the observations of other family members. For adults also, the input of family members is often very helpful.

Don't be shocked if the practitioner wants to talk to your spouse or friends. This is also helpful in cases where results have been difficult to attain and the practitioner needs a fresh perspective.

Take the medicine

Believe it or not, patients occasionally go through the trouble and expense of seeing a homeopathic practitioner and then, for one reason or another, do not take the medicine. If you forget how you were supposed to take it, or, if problems arise and you're not sure what to do, or, if you have misgivings and feel uncomfortable about the treatment, then contact your practitioner. It is amazing how people will sometimes rely on the questionable advice of an acquaintance or relative instead of talking to their practitioner.

Avoid interfering substances

Some substances may interfere with homeopathic remedies and/or a person's reaction to them. The first and foremost is coffee. Coffee is not a food; it is not nutritive. Its effects are medicinal and drug-like, which is why so many people become addicted to it. The use of coffee often interferes with remedies and patients who refuse to discontinue its use reduce the probability that they will get results with homeopathy.

Camphor is another common antidote to remedies.

Camphor is found in medicated analgesic balms such as Ben Gay, Vicks, Tiger Balm, White Flower, etc. Other odoriferous medicated products with such things as eucalyptus are sometimes a problem.

Recreational drugs such as marijuana, cocaine, and the like are interfering substances. Prescription drugs with similar effects such as Valium and other mood-elevators may also interfere. Patients on such prescription drugs can often get results if remedies are given on a daily-dose basis. These patients can usually discontinue the drugs after they respond to the remedy.

Raw onions and garlic are medicinal and sometimes interfere with remedies. Mint is sometimes a problem. Dental work sometimes causes problems. General anesthesia will often cause a setback in therapy.

Does this mean that all these things will interfere with treatment in any patient taking any remedy? Does it mean that no other things will interfere? The answer to both these questions is no. Everyone is different — that's the whole point with homeopathy. Some people get results regardless of their habits and life-style, while others, like the patient in the story opening this chapter, are more easily disturbed.

It's often hard, however, to tell in advance which substances will interfere with which patients. Since the above mentioned substances interfere with treatment in many patients, it is prudent to avoid them for best results.

The bottom line

The bottom line for results in homeopathy is straight forward. Make a commitment to yourself to stick with it. Work with your practitioner. Make a few reasonable life-style changes if needed. Avoid interfering substances. Take the remedy as directed.

Chapter 10

Special Situations

My wife, Ming, an acupuncturist who also practices homeopathy, got a call one day from a patient. The person to be treated was not her, but her friend's cat.

It seems the cat, a 12 year old female, had been diagnosed with lymphoma. It had all started about six months earlier when the cat lost its appetite, weight, and energy and started losing fur in "big gobs." Subsequent blood samples, x-ray, and veterinary exam resulted in the diagnosis. "It has a lump that can be felt growing in the gut; the lump was not there three months ago."

The cat was described as being very fastidious. It would not use the cat box unless it was fresh nor would it eat from a dirty bowl.

The cat was very chilly. It would sit in the sun for long periods or, if the sun was not out, it would curl up under the covers. It was very restless, constantly changing positions and moving about.

In recent months, the cat had been very possessive It didn't like other cats around. It had increased thirst but little appetite. It often vomited after eating.

Ming recommended homeopathic Arsenicum.

We heard intermittently about the cat from the patient. The cat responded quickly to the remedy, the lump disappeared, normal appetite returned, and it became its former playful self. Now, a few years later, the cat is still alive and well.

Pregnancy

All homeopathic remedies of 6X potency or higher are completely safe for anyone, including both mother and fetus. In fact, these medicines are probably the only truly safe therapy which exists for use in pregnancy.

Pregnancy is a dynamic state in which great changes take place in a short period of time. Perhaps it is this dynamism that makes pregnant women very responsive to homeopathic medicines. Not only can chronic problems of the mother be addressed but problems related to pregnancy can also resolve.

I have seen breech babies turn, premature contractions stop, vomiting of pregnancy resolve, and many other changes in pregnant women treated homeopathically.

Homeopathy is also safe and effective during labor and childbirth. Many midwives and physicians throughout the world use homeopathic remedies exclusively, with great success, in managing all kinds of labor-related problems.

For example, I have seen women who were experiencing painful labors calm down after a few homeopathic pellets melted under their tongue. They said it wasn't like a drug-induced state, but that after the remedy they could tolerate the pain and weren't so irritable.

Children

Homeopathy is safe for all ages, from newborn to old age. Children respond well to homeopathy. Nursing babies are sometimes treated by giving the remedy to the mother.

Children, like pregnant women, are in a dynamic, changing state, which is probably why they respond so well to remedies. Children raised in a homeopathic household often grow up never having taken an antibiotic.

The parents must learn to trust the wisdom of the body. For example, fevers are a response to disease, not a disease in themselves. It is not necessary or desirable to suppress most fevers. Instead, it is a good idea to know what is causing the fever (disease diagnosis), but then to treat the patient homeopathically. For the vast majority of childhood illnesses associated with fevers, the patient can be treated homeopathically with confidence.

There are a few illnesses where most homeopathic practitioners recommend conventional treatment. These are life-threatening illnesses, often requiring hospitalization, where conventional care yields good results. Bacterial spinal meningitis is a good example.

Most common problems that are routinely treated with conventional medications can be treated easily with homeopathy. Ear infections, for example, rarely need antibiotics.

Children with emotional and behavior problems often respond dramatically to homeopathic care. In fact, most of the time, the first change we look for in children is a positive change in behavior, even though their main complaint may be totally unrelated.

Home health

Manufacturers of homeopathic medicines sell home-health kits. These kits contain thirty to fifty commonly indicated remedies and a few lotions. Instructional books often accompany these kits.

Using homeopathic home-health kits is a time honored tradition. Family members with common complaints such as

coughs, colds, diarrhea, and vomiting can often be successfully treated with minimal training. However, treating patients
with chronic, often lifelong, illnesses requires years of training
and experience to get good results. Persons undergoing
treatment from a practitioner must not take other homeopathic
remedies without first consulting their practitioner.

It is not difficult to learn the basics of homeopathy for
home use. There are numerous good books on the subject.
Many cities have classes in homeopathy, often oriented
towards home care. (For both books and class information
see the Resources section in *Appendix 3.*)

Treating family members and friends with everyday
complaints is both fun and educational. Many people find the
experience gives them a sense of self-confidence and freedom
from an often intrusive medical system. It is rewarding to see
these problems resolve quickly and with little expense.

Through practice and experience, home prescribers
will improve their skills. There is no danger of a toxic reaction
to the remedies. The warning signs of more serious medical
conditions are usually presented in the various introductory
books on homeopathic home-health.

Remember that it is not necessary to treat every little
ache and pain of life. Trust the body's ability to heal itself.
Even very healthy people get occasional colds and other
minor problems.

Animals

The veterinary use of homeopathic remedies is an
interesting confirmation of the universality of the homeopathic response.

In conventional medicine, medicines are tested in
animals to determine the effects and toxic reactions. Then the
medicines can eventually be used in trials on people.

In homeopathy, just the opposite occurs. Provings are done on people. In this way, the subtle effects on thinking, emotions, and general symptoms (chilliness vs. warmth, thirst, etc.) can be determined.

Amazingly, these same indications brought out on people have been shown to apply to animals. Observant owners can often tell these features in their pets. It is actually similar to observing changes in pre-verbal children.

Animals suffering from illness may desire attention, want to be alone, or may be irritable and snappish. If chilly, they lay in the sun, if warm on the cold tiles. It is easy to tell if they are hungry, thirsty, restless, or calm.

Pet owners can learn to take care of their pets. Also, there are a growing number of veterinarians who specialize in homeopathy.

Veterinary homeopathy is especially interesting and useful because the distance between generations in animals is relatively short. In this way, veterinary homeopaths can observe familial tendencies, the effects of immunizations, and the effects of remedies from one generation to the next. Perhaps these observations made by homeopathic vets will eventually prove applicable to people.

The fact that homeopathic medicines work beautifully on animals using the indications brought out on humans is fascinating. It speaks to the universality of the homeopathic response as well as the fundamental unity of life. Perhaps this is what many pet owners are referring to when they say their pets are people, too.

Candida

Candida albicans is a type of yeast that can cause problems in humans. It is found as *thrush* in young babies mouths, can cause a bright red diaper rash, and is responsible for many complications of immunosuppressed patients.

It has also been implicated as a cause of yeast overgrowth especially in patients who have been treated with antibiotics. A diagnosis of candida infection is frequently made for patients with many symptoms such as food intolerances, fatigue, irritability, mood swings and the like.

Patients often ask of homeopathic practitioners, "Do you treat candida?" The simple answer to this is, "No. We treat patients who may have candida, but we do not treat candida."

From the point of view of homeopathy, candida is a disease diagnosis. The usual disease-oriented treatment includes taking an antifungal agent, such as Nystatin, to kill the yeast, and dietary changes. Whereas many patients benefit from these changes, the disease often recurs when they stray from the therapeutic diet.

There is no need in homeopathy for a specific candida treatment. The homeopathic approach treats the patient as a whole with one of a great many homeopathic remedies. A healthy patient is not susceptible to candida infections and will recover without specific disease treatment.

It is a common misunderstanding that once a diagnosis has been made, a specific disease treatment is mandatory. Over the years, patients with all kinds of disease diagnoses, even patients in whom the diagnosis is unclear, have benefited from homeopathic treatment.

Hormone replacement, menopause, and osteoporosis

Hormone replacement therapy is appropriate in a wide range of diseases involving damaged glands. For example, thyroid hormone replacement is well-indicated in a patient with a surgically removed or radioactively impaired thyroid gland. Likewise, in a patient with juvenile diabetes whose pancreas can no longer produce insulin, insulin replacement is lifesaving. Homeopathy can help these patients, but it is unlikely that their need for at least some hormone replacement will ever be gone.

The situation with menopausal women is entirely different. Menopause is a natural transition in life. A healthy woman with a healthy diet and proper exercise should pass through menopause with minimal discomfort and live to a ripe old age without hormone replacement.

The current trend in medicine is to give hormone replacement at the first signs of menopause as indicated by decreasing hormone levels on lab work. This reflects an empty rationality. Menopause is no more a disease than puberty is a disease. In homeopathy, we do not treat the lab work, we treat the patient. Menopausal women experiencing discomfort with menopause are treated as unique individuals the same way all patients are treated with homeopathy. Homeopathy has an excellent record of treating women through this transitional time without the use of exogenous hormones.

A number of natural plant hormone-like substances are promoted as alternatives to synthetic hormone re-placement. These may be preferable in many instances to synthetic replacement, but they still reflect a disease-oriented approach to what is, in reality, a natural process.

Hormone replacement is also promoted as a preven-tive measure for bone loss. Studies have shown that calcium loss in the body is primarily associated with certain life-style factors. Among these are included excess ingestion of meat, coffee, and alcohol. Also associated is a lack of proper exercise and inadequate calcium intake.

It's true that women with a strong family history of osteoporosis occurring in relatively young female members of their family may be at high genetic risk for this problem. Such patients, while a small minority, may indeed benefit from hormone replacement. Even in these patients, hormone replacement is only one option and must be weighed against the potential risks of treatment.

Chapter 11

Homeopathy and Conventional Medicine

Once upon a time there was a man who had a job sitting on tacks.

He went to his regular doctor. "My rear end hurts," he lamented. "Can't you give me something for it?"

The doctor gave him some pain medicine. Over time, the dose gradually increased until the man no longer felt the pain of sitting on the tacks. In fact, he hardly even noticed his job, he was in such a drugged state.

Eventually his doctor died. He went to a new doctor. The new doctor realized that he was causing the problem through his work and said, "I won't give you pain medicine, you need to quit your job!"

Unable to bring himself to quit, the man wandered the streets in despair. Finally, he entered the office of a homeopath.

"Why don't you quit?" the homeopath asked.

"I can't," the man replied. "They need me, there is no one else who can do the job."

The homeopath realized this man's real problem was his delusion that he must do this work. He gave the man a remedy. "It will cure your sore rear end," he told the man.

As the man responded to the remedy he changed his outlook. He quit his job and found a new vocation in life.

At the follow-up appointment the man said, "The remedy didn't work. I had to quit my job."

"Does your rear end hurt?" the homeopath asked.

"No, of course not!" the man replied.

Although this story is fictional, it accurately contrasts homeopathy and conventional medicine. No one has a job sitting on tacks, but patients often make amazing changes while undergoing homeopathic treatment.

An over-medicated population

The average person in America today is over-medicated. Patients take huge quantities of powerful medications prescribed by conventional physicians for what are, in reality, minor complaints. These same patients then consume over-the-counter medicines in large amounts for every little ache and pain. Finally, perhaps out of guilt, many people have a veritable pharmacy in their homes of high-potency vitamins and herbs with which they attempt to undo all the bad effects of their previous over-medication.

It is my observation that conventional physicians know that they prescribe medicines which many patients do not truly need. Patients, however, insist on receiving some kind of medicine and powerful allopathic medicines are the only medicines which are considered acceptable for these physicians to prescribe.

Ignorance on the part of patients and aggressive marketing are the main causes of over-the-counter medication use. Patients are made to think that they should not experience any symptoms or discomfort in their lives. People tend to forget that most symptoms which they experience represent their body's response to the illness, not the illness

itself. By constantly suppressing their natural healing response they get progressively more ill over time.

Differing approaches

The acceptance of homeopathy does not mean the
rejection of conventional medicine.

The conventional approach is analytic. *Analysis* means
the separation of a whole into its parts. Conventional
medicine focuses on the parts: the organs, the cells, the
cellular components and the molecules. The goal is to
understand the microbiological, biochemical, or cellular basis
for a disease and to correct it on that level.

Homeopathy is synthetic. *Synthesis* means the combination of the parts to form a whole. It is concerned mostly
with the whole, and the various parts are viewed from this
perspective. The goal is to understand the response of the
patient as a whole and to apply medicines based on that
understanding to stimulate the self-healing mechanism.

The whole is much greater than the sum of the known
parts. That's why conventional medicine, with its steadily
increasing knowledge of the parts, still falls far short of the
homeopathic perspective.

What this translates to in the practical world is that the
patients of homeopathic practitioners rarely require any
medicine other than homeopathic remedies when ill. There
do, however, exist health problems for which homeopathic
practitioners recommend conventional treatment.

Where to use conventional care

Conventional care is recommended for many urgent
problems that require immediate control of the disease for the
preservation of life or limb. Medical problems included here
are such things as life-threatening infectious diseases (such as

bacterial spinal meningitis), myocardial infarction, hypertensive crisis, and the like.

In the past, homeopathy was widely used for treating patients with these conditions. Homeopathy made its reputation in the nineteenth century with outstanding success in devastating epidemic infectious diseases such as cholera and typhoid.

Currently, the allopathic treatment is easier to apply and is efficient in saving lives and preventing permanent injury in patients with many of these immediately life-threatening problems.

I don't have an exact list of what diseases I recommend conventional treatment for. It depends on the patient, their disease, and situation in life. Suffice to say that I recommend conventional treatment for surprisingly few patients.

Antibiotic overuse

The treatment of bacterial infectious disease with antibiotics is one of the strengths of allopathic medicine. Due to the lack of any alternatives in allopathy, antibiotics are overused. With many patients, the more antibiotics they take, the more they need. It's a kind of vicious cycle where the immune system gets progressively less effective in resisting infections.

This overuse has also resulted in the development of "superbugs" — microorganisms resistant to antibiotics — and may be a cause of candida yeast overgrowth and associated fatigue syndromes.

Patients using homeopathy as their primary healthcare need antibiotics only occasionally, if at all. This represents a practical preventive solution to this developing problem of antibiotic resistance. Homeopathy also has potential value in the treatment of patients with infections caused by antibiotic resistant organisms.

Surgery

Surgery is another conventional modality sometimes needed. There exist many conditions, both medical and traumatic, which are best treated surgically. Homeopathy has been used successfully in preventing many surgeries but will not always suffice in a truly appropriate surgical condition.

If you get run over by a truck, clearly you'll need surgical care. Other conditions are not always so clear. For example, if an appendicitis is suspected, a remedy should be started while the patient is on the way for surgical evaluation. Surprisingly, a greater than expected number of these cases will resolve without surgery.

Many thousands of children get tubes placed in the ears for recurrent infections. My personal experience is that only very few of these children need such surgery if they get homeopathic care.

As with antibiotics, surgery tends to be overused. This is especially true in many gynecological conditions where there is no urgency to the surgery, the condition is not life-threatening, and yet surgery is performed without any attempt at healing.

Conventional medications

There are many conventional medications which should not be abruptly discontinued just because a patient decides to pursue homeopathic therapy. There are too many examples to list here, but the general idea is that if you have been controlling a disease with medication, it's not safe to abruptly stop the medication. It may be necessary to begin homeopathy and then wean the allopathic medicines, if possible, as the patient recovers. Homeopathy can still be of benefit to those patients who require certain medications which can not be safely discontinued.

One simple example is that of asthma. Many asthmatic patients control their asthma with medications. I usually start them on homeopathy and decrease their conventional medications as they respond.

A gray area

There is no distinct boundary as to exactly where the interface between homeopathy and conventional medicine lies. In many situations it depends on the experience of the practitioner and the desires of the patient. My personal experience is that most patients can be treated homeopathically. Conventional medicine and surgery should be reserved for certain patients and conditions of clear need.

The need for conventional medicine or surgery is not a failure. The heart of all forms of healthcare is the welfare of the patient.

Chapter 12

Homeopathy and Alternative Therapies

"I'm feeling fantastic!" one of my patients told me at a recent follow-up appointment. *"You see, I went to the 'Holistic Expo' and bought some herbal weight loss pills. I just started them ten days ago and my energy is wonderful.*

"I didn't want to tell you before I started them because I knew you'd tell me not to take them," she added.

It's true, I would have advised her to hold off on starting anything new. These herbal formulas help many people, but everyone is different. That's the whole point with homeopathy; patients must be treated as individuals.

This patient had been doing well on her remedy. Her last few menstrual periods had been the best in many years, they were on time and with few symptoms.

"Well," I said, *"since you already started it, let's see what happens. Maybe it will be fine with your remedy, maybe not. There's no way to tell without trying."*

Her next follow-up was six weeks later.

"I quit the herbal pills," she confided. *"I had the worst period in a long time. Also I gained five pounds."*

Now that she is off the herbs, her remedy should start acting again. Eventually, when her health has stabilized, *trying such pills probably won't throw her so out of balance. But, on the other hand, she also will not feel the need to try them.*

Alternative therapy

It is a misnomer to refer to homeopathy as an alternative therapy. It only appears alternative in that the conventional system is overused. It is no more alternative than the spherical earth view was an alternative to the flat-earth view in the fifteenth century. Homeopathy is not an optional outlook, but instead a more comprehensive one.

Likewise, practitioners of other alternative therapies prefer the use of another term, such as natural or complementary medicine, to distinguish their approach.

This section will discuss the compatibility of various non-conventional approaches to therapy or healthcare with homeopathy. Many systems, even though natural, interfere with the action of remedies and need to be avoided while undergoing treatment.

Holistic medicine

Holistic medicine is poorly defined. It is supposed to mean an approach which treats the whole person. Homeopathy is an excellent example of a truly holistic approach in that it does treat the whole person.

The problem is that holistic medicine is often allopathic in character. Much of naturopathy, ayurveda, oriental medicine, and herbal medicine is allopathic in that it primarily treats the disease as opposed to the patient.

This is easily seen by going into a store selling natural medicines. The same formulas are sold to everyone with the same disease or condition, much like conventional medicines.

(This is true even for many formulations sold as homeopathic medicines.)

This disease-oriented approach is not necessarily bad, but, as the case above illustrates, it does not take individual variation into account. In spite of this, these natural modalities are often preferable to conventional medicine because the treatments are usually safer and less toxic.

Naturopathy

Naturopathy is not the same as homeopathy. Naturopaths use a wide range of therapies to treat patients, one of which is homeopathy. A given naturopathic physician, however, may or may not be well-trained in homeopathy.

Accredited naturopathic education consists of a four year curriculum of traditional naturopathic courses as well as conventional diagnosis, obstetrics, minor surgery and the like. Graduates of the accredited institutions are well-rounded physicians and are eligible for licensure in those states which license naturopathic physicians. Unfortunately, there are also some non-accredited institutions which give degrees but have much lower standards. Graduates from these schools are not eligible for licensure anywhere in the US.

Despite the fact that virtually all naturopathic therapies are natural, not all are compatible for use simultaneously with homeopathy. Therapies such as therapeutic diets, fasting, massage, hydrotherapy, spinal manipulation (chiropractic and osteopathy), exercise, and many forms of physical therapy are compatible with homeopathy. These modalities do not force changes in the system.

Other modalities sometimes used by natural health practitioners, including naturopaths, are discussed below.

Nutrition

Proper nutrition is one of the pillars of good health. Most health conscious people today have a reasonable idea of what constitutes a proper diet. People need to eat simple, natural foods with adequate variety and in adequate amounts. They should avoid over-processed foods and non-food items. Quantities of rich foods, fats, meats, sugar, and the like are deleterious to health.

Beyond these straightforward guidelines, nutritional needs become very individual. Everyone's system is somewhat different. Some people don't tolerate certain foods which others thrive on. Some have allergies or intolerances which cause significant health effects such as recurring ear infections, asthma, or eczema in children. Often no medicine is needed at all, they just need to remove milk, or some other common offender, from their diet.

These individual variations are important in choosing a homeopathic remedy. Patients needing certain remedies often have food cravings or intolerances that are characteristic for that remedy.

Homeopathy in general does not insist on certain diets or nutritional therapy for those undergoing treatment, although specific patients may be advised to avoid or to encourage certain foods. Most practitioners observe that when patients respond to a remedy, they tend to desire a healthier diet spontaneously.

Vitamins

Many people advocate the use of vitamins and mineral supplements for the prevention of disease. The action of these supplements in the body varies depending on the dose in which they are taken.

Taken in smaller doses, vitamins act more as foods. In this range, close to their natural levels in foods, they are simply food supplements, supplying important dietary factors which, for one reason or another, a person may not be getting from their diet. Taken in very large doses, these same vitamins act more as medicines. For the most part they are non-toxic and safe, but they are medicines none-the-less. These large doses force shifts in the biochemical pathways of the body thereby giving relief in many conditions.

Such large doses of vitamins may be incompatible with homeopathy. Patients on these large doses find that their ability to respond to remedies is decreased. This is because the forced changes in the system may go contrary to the direction which the natural healing processes wish to go. As a result, the natural healing is thwarted.

This is not to say that vitamins are bad or in some way undesirable. It just means that while undergoing homeopathic treatment some patients need to downgrade their nutritional support to more natural levels.

Herbal medicines

Herbs may be compatible or incompatible with homeopathy depending on the herb and the patient. Many patients are so sensitive that even foods such as raw onions and garlic have a medicinal effect which will interfere with the patient's response to homeopathic remedies.

If an herbal medicine is being taken for its health effects there is a high likelihood that its action will interfere with a patient's response to homeopathic remedies. Marketing strategies on the part of herbal companies try to downplay the medicinal effects of herbs. It is true that many herbs also have nutritional properties, but most herbs and herbal combinations are sold and consumed for their medicinal effects.

Herbal teas which are consumed as beverages are often mild and do not interfere with remedies. Mint tea is one exception which may interfere.

Patients undergoing homeopathic therapy only occasionally need some other therapy at the same time. There are a few herbs that I sometimes recommend to patients, but for the most part, concurrent use of herbal medicines should be avoided. Patients can discuss specific questions with their practitioner.

Acupuncture

Acupuncture is the well-known system of oriental healing. Unfortunately, it may not mix well with homeopathy. I don't really know why this is. Some people undergoing acupuncture just don't seem to respond well to remedies while others do fine. My wife is an acupuncturist who also practices homeopathy and she also has found that many patients get better results if she keeps these modalities separate.

This is true for not only acupuncture with needles but also for moxa (heat) and Chinese herbs. Most forms of oriental massage do not interfere and can be used with homeopathy.

The mad rush

It comes as a surprise to many people that all forms of natural healing are not compatible if used simultaneously. Better results are usually obtained by doing one form of treatment at a time for its full benefit before trying something else.

Relax! In the mad rush to be healed, people waste much time and money by not giving whatever therapy they are doing a chance. True healing occurs from the inside out, in its own time, and cannot be forced.

Chapter 13

Homeopathic Remedies

A middle-aged woman with hyperthyroidism had been under my care for about four months. She was doing well. She was off her regular medication (called PTU) which she had taken for seven years. In the past, whenever she stopped the PTU, she became very ill within weeks; but now she had been off for the entire four months without symptoms. Her pulse, blood pressure, and other indicators of hyperthyroidism were all normal. She felt the best she had in years, emotionally stronger and with improved energy. It appeared that she was responding well to the remedy she was taking.

Her potency of this same remedy had just gone up a few weeks before. Suddenly I got a call from her.

"Dr. Dooley," she said, "I've been doing terrible the past few weeks. It just gets worse and worse. My pulse is racing and I'm nervous as a cat. This is what always used to happen off my PTU."

She came to the office and I reviewed her case. It just didn't make sense. There was no reason in my experience why she should be doing poorly. It appeared that the remedy had just stopped working.

She had not started any herbs or other medications which often interfere with remedies. She had not been drinking coffee. Her remedy had been properly stored and kept away from noxious fumes, direct sunlight, and other damaging factors.

Her old symptoms had started to return just a few days after starting the new potency of her remedy. The only conclusion I could come up with was that the remedy, when it arrived via UPS to her door from the manufacturer, had been somehow antidoted in route or improperly prepared.

After examination I concluded it was medically safe to wait for a few days while a new bottle of that same potency of the remedy was sent. She was skeptical but did not want to go back to PTU or to drink radioactive iodine (the next medical treatment in line for her).

Sure enough, when the new bottle arrived from the same manufacturer, she started on it and was better in just a few days. Within a week she had regained her previous level of well-being.

At the present time, there is no way to objectively measure the activity or strength of a homeopathic remedy other than by the response of a patient to it. It is therefore important to purchase remedies from reliable sources and to care for them properly. In my experience, it is rare that a remedy is inactive at the time of purchase. As this case demonstrates, it does occasionally happen.

Sources

Any substance which can affect human health and well-being can be developed into a homeopathic remedy. Provings have been conducted on a wide range of materials which are now part of the homeopathic Materia Medica.

Many remedies are made from herbs, both toxic and non-toxic. Remedies are made from minerals as benign as sodium chloride (common table salt), as deadly as arsenic, and as precious as gold and platinum.

There are remedies made from animals and animal products; some from insects such as bees or ladybugs. Others from products as seemingly exotic as snake venom, spider venom, or dog's milk.

Remedies can also be made from disease products and agents such as bacteria and scabies.

Regardless of the source of the remedy, it must be prescribed for the patient according to its homeopathic indications for good results. Each remedy must be made by the manufacturer in exactly the same manner as the substance used in the original provings. The final product will then reliably retain the known homeopathic indications as established in the provings.

Appearance

Each remedy is prepared in potency, as described in earlier chapters, so as to be non-toxic and yet to retain its unique homeopathic properties. As it is progressively diluted, the remedy quickly becomes a clear liquid. This clear liquid is then put onto small sugar pellets.

Homeopathic remedies therefore usually appear simply as small white pellets packaged in vials. The size of the pellets is not important. It's helpful to remember that the actual medicine is the tincture placed on the pellets, not the pellets themselves.

You can't tell one remedy from another by looking at the pellets. The label on the vial will tell the name of the remedy and its potency.

Labeling requirements

The U.S. Food and Drug Administration (FDA) requires that all over-the-counter medications have indications printed on the label. The reader of this book understands by now that there do not exist specific disease indications for homeopathic remedies. A patient with a given disease may need a single remedy out of hundreds. Likewise, a given remedy may be indicated for patients with one of many diseases found throughout the body.

In order to comply with FDA regulations, homeopathic manufacturers choose a common complaint for which a given remedy is indicated in many patients and place that indication on the label. This is often a source of confusion. For example, a homeopathic remedy prescribed for a male patient may be labeled as indicated for menstrual cramps. Or a patient whose main complaint is neurological might get a remedy labeled as indicated for diarrhea. Patients must realize that these so-called disease indications required by the FDA on homeopathic remedies are mostly irrelevant and should be ignored. For good results, all remedies should be taken only according to their homeopathic indications for the whole patient, not for the disease diagnosis on the label.

Prescription and unavailable remedies

In recent years the FDA has changed the status of some homeopathic remedies to prescription only. This is surprising to those familiar with homeopathy since all remedies were previously sold over-the-counter for over one hundred years without any reported problems.

The remedies now requiring prescriptions are those made from disease products. Persons familiar with the preparation of homeopathic medicines understand that it is literally impossible for these remedies to spread disease in any way.

The prescription status of these remedies is unnecessary and irrational, but at least they are still available.

Some other remedies have recently been made unavailable in the United States by the FDA. These include remedies made from controlled substances such as opium. Again, anyone familiar with even the most rudimentary basics of homeopathy understands that it is impossible for these remedies to be abused in any way. They are completely safe and are still available over-the-counter throughout the world except in the United States.

"Dr. Dooley," she said, "I'm sorry but I just get too large an emotional reaction to taking any drug like this, even in small doses. Many people in my family have had problems with drugs; my sister is finally clean now, and the thought of this really bothers me. Isn't there another remedy you can give me?"

The year was 1979 and I was in my naturopathic practice in southern Oregon. At that time, homeopathic opium was still available as an over-the-counter medicine here in the U.S.

"Mary," I said, attempting to explain. "When you take homeopathic opium there is not even one molecule of opium in the remedy. All that remains is a kind of imprint that opium makes on the diluting liquid.

"Think of it this way — you suffer from a disease state similar to that of opium toxicity. You have terrible constipation and are constantly falling asleep. Your pupils tend to be constricted and you are always too hot.

"Taking this homeopathic opium will cure you of this opium-like state from which you suffer.

"Unfortunately, there is no other remedy which will substitute. Homeopathic remedies can only be prescribed on their similar symptoms for results. This is true whether the original substance is an herb like chamomile, a poison like snake venom, a metal like aluminum, or a drug like opium. Your symptoms are similar to opium toxicity, not to anything else."

Mary thought about it and remembered the results we had achieved with her son's problems. She realized his symptoms had also been similar to the symptoms of the medicine that cured him. In the end, she took the remedy and benefited.

Combination remedies

Some homeopathic manufacturers produce a number of medicines called combination remedies which are sold to treat specific diseases and complaints. These products are combinations of many single homeopathic remedies in varied potencies mixed together. They are often sold as liquid drops as well as pellets and tablets.

Many patients find these products easy to use and effectively palliate various complaints. Whereas they sometimes relieve symptoms quickly and effectively, they rarely bring a patient to a level of health where the problems stop recurring. The problem is that when single remedies are mixed together it creates a completely new medicine. Until a proving is done on that particular combination of remedies, its unique homeopathic indications are not known and a truly curative response is rare.

They are used most frequently for common complaints such as teething in children, allergic symptoms, indigestion, etc.

Patients undergoing constitutional therapy with a homeopathic practitioner should strictly avoid these combination remedies, unless cleared in advance with their practitioner. Taking multiple homeopathic remedies commonly disrupts ongoing homeopathic care.

Care of the remedies
Homeopathic remedies are remarkably stable and retain their therapeutic properties for extended periods if properly cared for. Remedies should be kept in sealed containers away from strong odors, direct sunlight, excessive heat, and microwave. Many common household appliances generate large electromagnetic fields, so remedies should not be stored near these.

They should not be stored in the same areas as camphor containing products (Vicks, Ben Gay, Tiger Balm, etc.). Avoid exposure to x-ray machines at airports, although these detectors do not always disturb their action.

In recent years, homeopathic manufacturers have started putting expiration dates on the remedies. These dates appear to be arbitrary and irrelevant. If remedies are properly cared for, they have been known to retain their potency for a great many years.

How to take a remedy
Remedies are usually taken as dry pellets under the tongue. Two to four pellets usually constitutes one dose, although this may vary per the size of the pellets. The number of pellets taken at each dose is not as important as the frequency of repetition or the potency.

For example, taking four pellets per dose is usually not very different from taking two pellets per dose. But taking four pellets once a day is very different from taking two pellets twice a day. Finally, taking four pellets of 6C is entirely different from taking two pellets of 12C.

Confused? To make life simple, just take the remedy as instructed by the practitioner. If you're not sure what to do, just ask.

It's important to remember that the sugar pellets are not the medicine, the medicine is the dilution which has been used to medicate the pellets. It is best not to touch the pellets with your fingers. Just use the cap of the vial to dispense the pellets and pour the correct number under your tongue from the cap. If pellets fall on the floor, it is best to dispose of them.

Patients are sometimes instructed to put the pellets in water and stir the water before taking a teaspoonful as a dose. This process slightly changes the potency and effect of the remedy. It is occasionally referred to as *plussing*.

Chapter 14

Changing
Your View

For three years, Ming (my wife) and I ran a weekly clinic in Tijuana, Mexico. Here we provided healthcare, at no charge, to the local residents. It was located next to the municipal dump in a very poor "colonia" (neighborhood). The people living here supported themselves by working in the dump digging all day through garbage and filth, recycling anything of value.

For a long time we set up a little clinic every week in the bedroom of one family's home. Their house was made of old forklift pallets nailed together. There was scrap metal on the outside and cardboard tacked on the inside. The cardboard was painted blue. A piece of plastic incorporated into the scrap ceiling let in a pale light. There were carpet remnants thrown over the dirt floor. There was no plumbing or electricity, but a car battery powered a small black and white TV. A statue of the Virgin Mary rested above it. Cooking was done over an open fire pit on the side of the house. There was a crude outhouse in the rear of the house next to a smelly pigpen.

As the years went by, we became familiar with many families in the community. Hospitals and friends here in the

U.S. donated medicines and a service organization eventually built a small clinic for our use.

The conventional pharmacy of the little clinic grew and grew. The reason is, we hardly ever used it! The donated conventional medicines just sat there. We found we rarely needed any medicine other than homeopathic remedies for taking care of just about everything. We brought our own remedies every week in hundreds of small vials carried in a red tool chest and then dispensed what was needed in small envelopes.

It was a little sad to watch the conventional medicines, so kindly donated for our use, go bad on the shelves. Eventually, I started passing the donated medicines on to the local chapter of the Red Cross for use in their clinic.

Homeopathy is a wonderful asset in third world and relief-work settings. Our patients in the clinic didn't really understand homeopathy. They just went to the doctor and got some pills. The children liked taking them. People got well.

Homeopathy is a vast subject and this book is only a short introduction. Yet, if you've read the entire book, you now understand many of the basics of homeopathy and what makes it different. You can see that there's no other system of medicine quite like homeopathy. You can see how it is possible that people of all ages with many types of complaints can benefit from homeopathy, while, at the same time, homeopathy does not directly treat disease!

You can see how homeopathy, not relying on high-tech testing, saves money. And you can see how homeopathy is natural, how it works with the body to promote the innate self-healing mechanism.

You should also be able to understand why conventional medical studies, which compare uniform treatments for a given disease, are rarely of use in evaluating homeopathy. In homeopathy, there is no uniform treatment for a given disease, the treatment varies according to the patient.

Recently, however, there have been a few published studies where homeopathy was used appropriately. The results of these studies supported the efficacy of homeopathy and they are referenced in *Appendix 4.*

So what now?

Some readers at the end of this book may find that they are ready to go. They feel they have understood the message of the book, they agree with it, and look forward to using homeopathy to improve their lives. Such people often find that homeopathy is an outlook they already had, but never expressed.

Interested persons will find the Resources section in *Appendix 3* useful. In it are recommended books, book dealers, organizations, manufacturers, and referral sources for practitioners.

Other readers may not be quite so comfortable. Perhaps they are not sure why. Perhaps they are skeptical or have lots of questions. It is common to have such reservations about something that is different, especially when one's health is the issue.

The reality is, changing one's outlook requires more than simple intellectual understanding. Although wanting to change is usually the first step, experience is often necessary before the change becomes a part of one's view.

Falling off the edge

In the early sixteenth century, European sailors and discoverers took the bold step of exploring the uncharted waters of the world. But simply understanding that the earth was a sphere did not calm their fears. The experience of successfully navigating the earth's oceans without falling off the edge was required to convince themselves that it was so.

These sailors had been raised with the belief that the earth was flat. Many had relatives who had sailed off the edge, that is, set out across the seas never to return. So, in spite of themselves, when they personally set off to challenge this flat-earth dogma, they found their knees shaking, their hearts pounding, and cold sweat forming on their brows.

After a voyage or two they found they had changed. They now not only intellectually knew the earth was a sphere, but, through their experience, this knowledge had become a part of them.

Homeopathy may be new to you, but to many others it is well-known. Their knowledge and experience is available to guide you, should you choose to pursue it.

Personal responsibility

You and you alone are responsible for your health. No amount of expert consultations can change this simple fact. The opinions of experts can help in your decision making, but, in the end, it is you who will live with the consequences of those decisions.

Adopting the holistic view of homeopathy does not limit any healthcare choices. On the contrary, understanding homeopathy encompasses conventional medicine while opening a new world of healthcare possibilities.

The final word

At this point in my life, I've worked in a variety of healthcare settings: from my naturopathic family practice in Oregon, to the hospital residency, to the slums of Tijuana. I've done rotations in hospital wards in Calcutta, India, and was director of a small rural hospital emergency department here in California for a number of years.

There are many interesting and useful therapies in this world, some natural, some not. But I have yet to find anything which takes the place of homeopathy.

At best, homeopathy represents a new branch of science that, when better understood, will open new vistas throughout the biological sciences as it does in healthcare.

At worst, homeopathy is a harmless placebo demonstrating that much of conventional medicine is unnecessary and harmful.

My direct experience with homeopathy is such that I say with confidence, of the above two possibilities, the first, the best scenario, is the correct one.

Appendix 1

Potentization of medicines

All medicines prepared by potentization start as a solution of established chemical strength. Then, one part of the solution is added to 99 parts of a diluent (water and/or alcohol) and the dilution is thoroughly succussed (vigorously agitated by shaking). This new dilution is called the 1C potency because it is a 1:100 dilution of the original solution (C standing for centesimal).

Then the 1C potency is further diluted by taking one part and adding 99 parts of a diluent. Again, the new dilution is succussed. The new dilution is called the 2C potency because it has been prepared by a 1:100 dilution performed twice. Hence, the actual strength of the 2C potency is 1:10,000 of the original solution (1/100 of 1/100). This is more clear if you study the illustration on the opposing page.

In a like manner, the succeeding potencies are all prepared (3C from the 2C, 4C from the 3C, etc.). It should be emphasized that the medicine must be thoroughly agitated after each dilution. If properly diluted and agitated, the medicines retain their ability to cause a homeopathic response even in the high potencies (high dilutions). If not properly agitated at each step, the medicine loses its homeopathic medicinal properties through the diluting process.

There is another system of potentization in which the dilution factor is 1:10 (a decimal dilution), instead of 1:100 (a centesimal dilution as discussed above). The overall process is otherwise the same and the resulting dilutions are referred to as 1X, 2X, 3X, etc.

The very high potencies are abbreviated by the use of the letter M. Hence, 1,000 C is usually referred to as 1M, 10,000 C as 10M, etc.

Potencies of nearly every strength might be used in the course of homeopathic treatment. For example, in the course of a day a homeopathic practitioner may prescribe low potencies, such as 6X, or high potencies, such as 10M, depending on the needs of the patients.

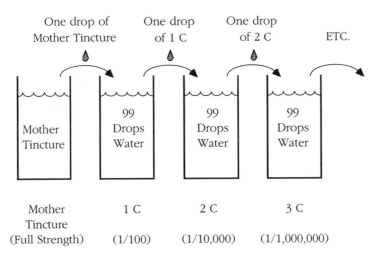

The process of potentization. Succussion (vigorous agitation by shaking) must be performed after each dilution step.

Appendix 2

A sample remedy

As an example of how a medicine is described in the Materia Medica, common white arsenic, called Arsenicum Album, is presented in part. The indications shown below represent some of the things which can be caused and cured by arsenic.

ARSENICUM ALBUM

MIND: Oversensitive, fastidious, fault finding. Anxious. Despair of recovery. Terrible fear of death. Worse at night. Restless, constantly changing position. Suspicious. Miserly, malicious, selfish. Irritability. Fear of robbers. Sees ghosts day and night.

HEAD: Aching, better cold. Restless, in constant motion. Scalp sensitive, cannot brush hair.

NOSE: Thin, watery, excoriating discharge. Cold sores in nose. Cannot bear sight or smell of food. Sneezing with coryza.

FACE: Pale, anxious, sunken. Cold sweat. Old look, in children.

STOMACH: Cannot bear sight or smell of food. Intense, unquenchable thirst. Drinks little and often. Craves ice cold water. Nausea, retching and vomiting. Desires sour things, brandy, coffee, milk.

SLEEP: Disturbed, anxious, restless. Shocks on dropping to sleep. Dreams of death, full of care, sorrow, and fear. Talks in sleep.

Get the general idea? The Materia Medica continues on through the various body systems, general symptoms, and modalities (things that make better and worse).

The Materia Medica lists a large number of symptoms which *might* be found in a person needing a given remedy. Most patients will only have *some* of the possible characteristic symptoms.

For example, most patients requiring Arsenicum Album are not miserly and suspicious, although these qualities will sometimes be found in patients needing the remedy.

Appendix 3

Resources

Recommended books:
Homeopathy in general
Homeopathy: Medicine for the New Man
By George Vithoulkas

Discovering Homeopathy: Medicine for the 21st Century
By Dana Ullman, MPH

The Patient Not the Cure
By Dr. Marjorie Blackie

Home treatment books
Homeopathic Medicine at Home
By Maesimund Panos, MD and Jane Heimlich

Everybody's Guide to Homeopathic Medicines
By Stephen Cummings, MD and Dana Ullman, MPH

The Complete Homeopathy Handbook
By Miranda Castro

Homeopathic Medicine for Children and Infants
By Dana Ullman, MPH

Where to buy books
Most large book stores and health food stores carry a few books on homeopathy. For a better selection, try one of the specialty mail order houses, a few of which are mentioned

here. Get one of their catalogues for a huge listing of homeopathic books, including many other home treatment books as well as advanced books.

Homeopathic Education Services
2124 Kittredge St.
Berkeley, CA 94704
(800) 359-9051(orders)
(510) 649-0294

Minimum Price Homeopathic Books
250 H Street
P.O. Box 2187
Blaine, WA 98231
(800) 663-8272

Where to buy remedies

Many natural food stores, health food stores, and traditional pharmacies carry homeopathic remedies. Just check the phone book and call around. They can also be ordered over the phone and shipped to your home. The numbers of some of the more common manufacturers and suppliers are listed below.

Standard Homeopathic
210 West 131st St.
P.O. Box 61067
Los Angeles, CA 90061
(800) 624-9659
Dolisos
3014 Rigel Ave.
Las Vegas, NV 89102
(800) 365-4767

Boiron
> 98C West Cochran St.
> Simi Valley, CA 93065
> (800) BLU-TUBE

Boericke and Tafel
> 2381 Circadian Way
> Santa Rosa, CA 95407
> (800) 876-9505

Homeopathy Overnight
> 4111 Simon Rd.
> Youngstown, OH 44512
> (800) 276-4223

Luyties Pharmacal Company
> 4200 Laclede Ave.
> St. Louis, MO 63108
> (800) 325-8080

Organizations

There are many professional and public homeopathic organizations.

The main one that can help you is:
> The National Center for Homeopathy (NCH)
> 801 North Fairfax Street, Suite 306
> Alexandria, VA 22314
> (703) 548-7790

The NCH has directories of practitioners, classes, workshops, seminars, and other services. They teach homeopathic courses in the summer. Their monthly newsletter is informative and up-to-date. Schools and other educational programs advertise in their newsletter. The NCH sponsors study groups around the country.

Membership in the NCH is inexpensive. You don't need to be a member to give them a call and inquire about practitioners, classes, and the like.

Another good organization is:
> International Foundation for Homeopathy (IFH)
> 2366 Eastlake Ave. E
> Seattle, WA 98102
> (206) 324-8230

The IFH also has a newsletter, teaches classes, and has information you may need. Like the NCH, IFH membership is reasonably priced.

These are the two main national organizations for the general public. You may also contact the national professional organizations for information and practitioner information. There are too many organizations to place them all in this appendix. Check with the NCH for information about your state or local organizations.

Practitioners

The primary ways to find practitioners are word of mouth, the yellow pages (either under Homeopaths or Physicians, homeopathic), or by referring to a directory. The NCH (see above) maintains a national directory and a few phone calls can usually help you find a practitioner in your area.

Appendix 4

Research studies

Ferley JP, Smirou D, D'Adhemar D, Balducci F., "A Controlled Evaluation of a Homeopathic Preparation in the Treatment of Influenza-like Syndromes." *Br J Clin Pharmacol* 1989;27:329-35.

Fisher P, Greenwood A, Huskisson EC, Turner P, Belon P., "Effect of Homeopathic Treatment on Fibrosistis (Primary Fibromyalgia)." *Br Med J* 1989; 299:365-6.

Gibson RG, Gibson SL, MacNeill AD, Buchanan,WW., "Homeopathic Therapy in Rheumatoid Arthritis: Evaluation by Double-blind Clinical Therapeutic Trial." *Br J Clin Pharmacol* 1980; 9:453-9.

Jacobs J, Jimenez LM, Gloyd SS, Gale JL, Crothers D., "Treatment of Acute Childhood Diarrhea with Homeopathic Medicine: a Randomized Clinical Trial in Nicaragua." *Pediatrics* 1994; 93:719-25.

Kleijne J, Knipschld P, ter Riet G., "Clinical Trials of Homeopathy." *Br Med J*, 1991;302:326-323 (meta-analysis)

Reilly DT, Taylor MA, McSharry C, Aitchison T., "Is Homeopathy a Placebo Response? Controlled Trial of Homeopathic Potency, with Pollen in Hayfever as Model." *Lancet*, 1986; ii: 881-5.

Index

Purchasing Information

Additional copies of **Homeopathy: Beyond Flat Earth Medicine** may be purchased directly from:

Timing Publications
4095 Jackdaw St.
San Diego, CA. 92103
(619) 299-1140

PRICES

# of Books	Cost	Shipping/Handling
1	$9.00 per book	$3.00
2	$8.10 per book (10% off)	$4.00
3	$7.20 per book (20% off)	$5.00
4	$6.30 per book (30% off)	$5.50
5 (or more)	$5.40 per book (40% off)	$6.00+

Additional shipping: $.50 per book for each book over 5. Foreign orders: add 50% to the shipping charges.

California residents must add 7.75% sales tax to the cost of the books (before shipping charges are added.)

Orders must be prepaid in US funds only. Checks, money orders and credit cards accepted. Please include cardholder's name, type of card (Visa or Mastercard), card number, expiration date, and telephone number. Phone orders accepted.

California tax and shipping subject to change.
Allow 2 to 3 weeks for delivery.